HERE I STAND

The Former U.S. Surgeon General

Dr. M. JOYCELYN ELDERS *his Sister*

Speaks Out On The Problems Facing America Today

HIV
School Based Health Care
Adolescent Self-Esteem
Health Care Reform
What Concerned Citizens Can Do

COMPILED BY
CHESTER R. JONES

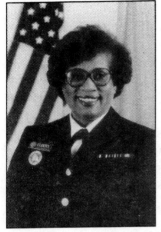

Dr. M. Joycelyn Elders has always been an outspoken advocate for health care, particularly for children and the elderly. In a series of speeches, recorded and compiled by her brother, Dr. Elders once again speaks out on the issues before America.

Born and raised in the tenant-farming days at Schaal, Arkansas, she joined the U.S. Army and graduated from medical school in the 1950's. Later she became the Director of the Arkansas Department of Health, and ultimately, Surgeon General of the United States.

Often controversial in her views, no one has accused her of being insincere in her observations on health care. She speaks out, loud and clear, and often to the amazement of her brother. "Here I Stand" focuses on her views .. unvarnished and with no apologies.

Chester R. Jones is a younger brother to Joycelyn Elders. Educated in the public schools of Arkansas, he received a Bachelor of Arts degree in Religion/Philosophy from Baker University in Baldwin, Kansas; a Master of Divinity degree from Gammon Theological Seminary in Atlanta, Georgia; and is ABD from Drew University in Madison, New Jersey. Rev. Jones received an honorary doctorate in humane letters from Philander Smith College in Little Rock, Arkansas. He currently serves as District Superintendent for the Pine Bluff District of the Little Rock Conference, United Methodist Church.

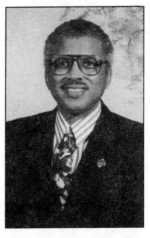

Dr. Jones has commented, "She raises difficult questions, and it has not been easy to be Dr. Elders' pastor and brother. So I am grateful that there is only one Joycelyn Elders in our family. I will venture to say, God blessed America by having only one like her in the country."

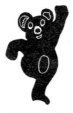

Printed in the United States of America

First Edition, 1997

Library of Congress Catalog Card Number: 97-069442
ISBN 0-9653996-1-3

CONTENTS

ACKNOWLEDGMENTS

I want to express my appreciation to Dr. Charles Donaldson, Vice Chancellor of the University of Arkansas at Little Rock; my secretary, Jan Stone, in the Pine Bluff United Methodist District; my brother-in-law Coach O.B. Elders; and my wife, Valarie Abbott Jones, attorney and conflict resolution facilitator.

Last, but certainly not least, my very special thanks to Dave and Ernie Wallis of Wallis and Wallis Advertising, Pine Bluff, for the technical assistance in the printing of this book.

Rev. Chester R. Jones

DEDICATED

To our father: Curtis Jones

And

The Children of The World

"Fear not, Stand firm, and See the salvation of the Lord" (Exodus 14:13)

FOREWORD

Here I Stand brings the point home. It is past time for us to take off the blinders and deal with the issues. America has a health care crisis on its hands with almost 38,000,000 of its citizens, most of whom are children, with little or no health care insurance. Dr. Elders states, "We see our children out in the ocean surrounded by the sharks of drugs, alcohol, homicide and suicide. We sit on the beach moralizing and talking about whose values should be taught, while our children drown. We have not addressed the needs and issues using up our children." This famous quotation from Dr. Elder's speech to the Global Gathering, sponsored by the General Board of Global Ministries of the United Methodist Church in Indianapolis, Indiana, gives a hint of the kind of hard hitting messages in this book.

In these powerful public speeches, Dr. Elders has persuaded many of us to open up discussion of once taboo subjects. These speeches will help you understand what Dr. Elders really said without the influence of slanted television or newspaper versions. In these speeches, she dare, in a manner unlike anyone else, to address the major health care issues.

Does she know of what she speaks? You bet! Dr. Elders has seen it all. She grew up in economic poverty. There was no silver spoon for her. Dr. Elders knows what poverty without intervention can do to good people who are otherwise sound. She speaks of the poor and the destructive effects of "The 5-H Club," ... healthlessness, homelessness, huglessness, hopelessness, and hunger. According to Dr. Elders, if we, as a nation, are to address welfare reform and the destructive effects of poverty, then "we have got to do more than offer rhetoric."

In 1987, then Governor Bill Clinton asked Dr. Elders to be the Director of the Arkansas Department of Health. In the words of Dr. Harry P. Ward, Chancellor of the UAMS College of Medicine, she remolded the health department into an active health service program by stimulating the formation of school based clinics, community centers, etc. Of most importance, she addressed the major issues of teenage pregnancy, childhood immunization, AIDS, maternal newborn care, access to care for the poor, teen violence, etc. In many cases, her positions and opinions caused controversy. In all cases, she opened the window. At least we have been debating the right subjects. (*Ward, Harry P. "Time in the Trenches." Editorial. UAMS Journal. Summer, 1993:2*)

Dr. Elders is bold in her attempts to incite reform of our health care thinking. There were those who characterized her work with the Arkansas Department of Health as a crusade mission. She called it a responsibility. No matter how we may view her work, one common theme seems central to whatever her discourse. If we are to change attitudes toward personal health care, our emphasis in medical care must shift to the prevention mode.

Finally, at the heart of this book is a caring crusader's cry for change in the way we view and deliver health care in America. Whenever Dr. Elders speaks — if we can put aside racism, sexism, — we can hear her assurance that "We can change if we choose to change." It is certainly clear that our present approach is not working. Dr. Elders offers more than just a radical approach to change; she offers hope. Although outspoken and passionate, Dr. Elders is dedicated to her mission. She advocates prevention and public health education as ways to make American healthy. It is her belief that Americans have a prime opportunity to take a critical look at our present health care situation. Dr. Elders says, "In order to meet the challenges of the twenty-first century, we must have a healthy America."

God Is Love

Chester R. Jones
Noahs of Ark Emmaus Walk #58
Table of Thomas

ONE
On Our Task at Hand
Where Should We Go from Here?

All Americans, regardless of geographic location, economic status, or race, may share in the joy and significance of recalling and acting upon the legacy of Dr. Martin Luther King, Jr.

Our task is to revitalize and keep alive the spirit and memory of our fallen leader and of the movement he helped begin. At the heart of that movement are the principles of racial equality and nonviolent social change.

In one of Dr. King's last and most radical addresses as head of the Southern Christian Leadership Conference, he raised the question: *Where do we go from here?* Let me share my vision and dream of some places we ought to go.

What Are Some of the Places Where We Ought to Go?

Dr. King had a three-point program.

1) The first part had to do with education and self-awareness. First and foremost we must go to school. We must educate ourselves to know that we are *somebody*. We are human beings made in God's image. And I say that's good!

However, you know as well as I that many of our bright young people don't think they are *somebody*. Therefore, they are selling themselves to drug addiction, teenage pregnancy, and violent gang behavior. We need to teach our bright young people to be *somebody*, to stay in school

1

and get a good education. If you think education is expensive, keep in mind that it is not half as expensive as ignorance. The slogan used to promote our black colleges is correct: *A mind is a terrible thing to waste.* Therefore, we must recommit ourselves to helping our young people stay in school and benefit from a good education.

2) The second part of Dr. King's program had to do with jobs and economic development. After we get a good education, we need places to work. Unemployment among our black young people is absolutely too high. Unemployment for the black young male population is almost five time that of white young males.

We in the black community must get back to the basics and develop a vital work ethic. Dr. King knew that people cannot reach their full potential unless they are economically strong. To become economically strong requires a great deal of discipline and sacrifice. Job creation and increasing minority business ownership will be tough objectives to achieve and require strong discipline.

Yet as Dr. M. Scott Peck says in his book *The Road Less Traveled:* "Life is a series of problems, and discipline is the basic tool required to solve life's problems."

Without discipline we can solve nothing. With total discipline we can solve any problem. What makes life difficult is that solving problems is painful. Yet it is only in meeting and solving problems that we grow mentally and spiritually. Only if we are willing to stumble now and then on the pathway to success will we ever reach our goals. A mistake should be viewed only as an occasional misstep. I always view mistakes as being positive, a lesson learned. A person with a perfect record, without any mistakes, is often a person who never took any risks.

3) The third part of Dr. King's program had to do with political awareness. He knew the importance of voter registration and running for office. To be productive citizens we must participate in the political arena.

We must go out and vote. But just participating in the political arena is not enough. We must develop a plan to address the problems that are still facing our people: poverty, homelessness, illiteracy, black-on-black crime, teenage pregnancy, drug abuse, HIV, and related concerns. I am sure if Dr. King were alive today he would find a way to bring us together again to address these issues and fight and march until the victory is won.

There are countless children trapped by poverty in rural areas and our inner cities. To fulfill Dr. King's dream, we must provide our young people with strong role models to help them stay in school, stay off drugs, and stay out of jail. We need job programs that will prepare uneducated and unskilled blacks to fill their share of the new jobs our society is creating daily. We need to work and develop economic opportunities and programs to transform our cities from battlegrounds into peaceful communities.

So where do we go from here? We must go into our prayer closets and make some hard choices. We must choose between education and ignorance, hard work and unemployment, freedom and jail, Morehouse (college) and the poorhouse, Philander Smith (college) and Tucker (state prison).

I am inspired by these lines:
People are unreasonable, illogical, and self-centered.
Love them anyway!
If you do good, people will accuse you of selfish, ulterior

motives.

Do good anyway!

If you are successful, you will win false friends and true enemies.

Succeed anyway!

The good you do today will be forgotten tomorrow.

Do good anyway!

Honesty and frankness make you vulnerable.

Be honest and frank anyway!

The biggest people with the biggest ideas can be shot down by the smallest people with the smallest minds.

Think big anyway!

People favor underdogs, but follow only top dogs.

Fight for some underdogs anyway!

What you spend your years building may be destroyed overnight.

Build anyway!

People really need help, but may attack you if you help them.

Help people anyway!

Give the world the best you have, and you'll get kicked in the teeth.

Give the world the best you have anyway!

Where Should We Go from Here?

We must make choices which lead us

- providing quality education for each and every citizen;
- toward cultivating a vital work ethic and assuring that all our people have access to productive jobs;
- toward promoting full participation in the political process and implementing comprehensive plans to improve the quality of life in our communities.

TWO
On HIV
Can We Get Where We Need to Go?

All of us know that we face significant challenges in the field of health care–especially in the fight against HIV. To address these challenges, we have organized committees and commissions in every state. We have formed groups to study what is needed in specific communities. We have engaged in scientific research. We have helped great numbers of people through education programs and prevention measures. And we have made genuine progress. However, we still must ask: *Can we get where we need to go from here?*

We are more than a dozen years into the HIV epidemic. More than 200,000 persons in the United States have been diagnosed with HIV/AIDS. While considerable progress has been made, the painful truth is that there is still no cure at hand and the disease is continuing to spread through all sections of the United States.

We are now seeing a change in the faces of those who have, and are acquiring, the disease. These faces belong to people of color, women, and babies. In fact, AIDS has become one of the leading causes of death among women of childbearing age.

We know where we need to go, so I ask again: Can we get there from here? The answer is a resounding *yes*, but it will take all of us working together–from the federal government to individuals. The federal government needs to admit that HIV is a major health problem. The government can allocate dollars for research and health care. If we can find millions to buy and build bombs to destroy human beings, certainly we must be willing to provide the funds required to preserve or save the lives of human beings. In addition to allocating funds, the federal government can establish necessary laws to protect all citizens. But federal agencies cannot work in isolation. They must join a coalition that includes state and local governments as well as community groups and religious organizations.

Many state and local agencies have acknowledged the fact that HIV is spreading, but they have not provided the assistance that is needed to face this challenging problem. Too many people are not receiving education or preventive information, and many go undiagnosed and untreated simply because state and local governments have given only lip service to the fight against HIV.

Community organizations have provided services to educate our citizens. They have sponsored numerous forums, workshops, and other forms of disseminating information. Churches and religious groups are gradually getting involved because they are faced with situations where family members of people with AIDS need counseling and other assistance to get through the crisis.

We see many individuals and groups working to combat HIV—but too often in isolation from each other. I ask again: Can we get where we need to go from here?

As a state health director I encountered many citizens who had their heads in the sand, people who refuse to acknowledge the problems of teen pregnancies and drug abuse, and—even worse—people who fail to see the relationships between teen pregnancies and drug abuse and the increase of HIV and sexually transmitted diseases. As a medical doctor who is well aware of the enormity of these problems and challenges, I am convinced that we *can* get where we need to go from here.

However, it requires that we build new and bold coalitions. No longer can we work in isolation. We must work together–from the federal government to individuals, from the health care providers to those involved in the administration of education and prevention programs.

I challenge every citizen, every health care worker, and every educator to make a commitment to make a difference. We have the *know-how*, we have the *resources* — all we need to do is make the commitment. We must communicate and work together cooperatively to form partnerships. Each of us has a role to play in responding to this crisis.

Can we not all agree that we share a common and urgent mission? That mission is not to change lives, but to save them.

Can We Get Where We Need to Go?

The answer is yes! if we:

- acknowledge that the problems of teen pregnancies and drug abuse are directly related to the sharp increase of HIV-related illness in people of color, women, and babies;

- allocate dollars for research and health care, and if we no longer work in isolation from one another but instead form new and bold coalitions between federal, state, and local governments, as well as community groups and religious organizations;

- recognize that our greatest need is not the know-how or financial resources — but the commitment to work together to win the battle against HIV.

7

THREE
On Adolescent Health
Can We make a Difference?

America was founded as a land of hope — a land in which the poor, the persecuted, and people seeking a better life could find refuge. It was founded on the belief that through education and hard work people could experience a full and prosperous life. And, for most of its people, this is true. More children are born healthy, achieve in school, have a high self-esteem and hope for the future, and are able to develop into productive members of society.

But for some, it is a different land. These people suffer from poor health, have limited education and few job skills, and face seemingly insurmountable obstacles to achieving self-sufficiency and productivity. And at the same time, the United States is facing a multitude of challenges which require that more and more of its people be productive participants in society.

Improved and consistent health care is one area that could substantially enhance the quality of life for many Americans. For a variety of reasons, however, too many citizens don't get the health care they need and deserve.

- For example, in 1990, about 12 percent of the GNP was spent on medical costs, yet only 2.9 percent of the GNP went to prevention programs. More than a third of the country's population, 100 million, is without adequate health insurance protection.

- Almost one-fourth of the pregnant women in this country get late or no prenatal care. Over half a million residents of rural counties, many of them in the South are without physicians who provide obstetric care.

8

The obstacles to self-sufficiency and productivity are further reflected in the statistics on the status of our young people–our future leaders. They are being overwhelmed by multiple interrelated problems.

For every one hundred children born today:

• fifteen will be born to households where no parent is employed;

• and twenty-five will depend on welfare for at least a portion of their childhood.

In addition, each year:
• more than 1.1 million girls, ages 10 to 19, become pregnant (12.4 percent of all births);
• over 2 million children are reported as abused or neglected;
• 2.5 million teenagers contract a sexually transmitted disease;
• more than one-half-million 12- to 17-year-olds try cocaine;
• approximately 1,800 youths are victims of homicide, and more than 2,000 adolescents take their own lives;
• according to the national Household Survey on Drug Abuse in 1988, 50 percent of 12 -to 17-year-olds have at least tried alcoholic drinks;
• approximately 12 adolescents a day are killed in alcohol-related injuries;

The plight of young black males is especially precarious. They are dying disproportionately from homicide (their leading killer), suicide (tripled since 1960), and drug abuse. They are over represented among high school dropouts and under represented on college campuses. In Arkansas, we have more young black men in prison than in college, and

9

that is not unique.

These statistics point to conditions that hold little hope of a "full and prosperous life" for a significant part of America's population. These are the children on whom we will depend for decisions in the twenty-first century.

While the impact of these problems is apparent in the loss of human potential, in the cost of governmental services, in the loss of productivity, and in increased costs to the private sector, the full scope of the causes and effects is not easily determined. They are intertwined and cannot be approached singly.

As a nation, we have begun to take some tentative steps toward addressing these issues. The (1991) Surgeon General's Goals for the Year 2000 challenge us to address several critical areas. These include:

- reducing instances of low birth weight from 6.9 percent to 5 percent and very low birth weight from 1.2 percent to 1 percent;

- reducing pregnancies among girls aged 17 and younger from 71.1 per 1,000 to no more than 50 per 1,000;

- increasing the percentage of students graduating from high school from 79 percent to 90 percent.

In addition, Congress has taken significant steps in recent years toward improving the health of women and children, beginning with the passage of SOBRA in 1986. OBRA 89 and OBRA 90 have continued to make improvements by:

- requiring increased coordination between WIC (Women, Infants and Children) and Medicaid;

- establishing new accountability procedures and increasing funding for Title V:

• expanding Head Start 26 percent in FY 91 by increasing funding by $400 million).

Revised federal health policies, targeting of financial resources, education, interagency cooperation, and private initiatives at the local level will all be key elements in improving the future. To be effective in meeting these challenges many partnerships are needed at all levels. Local, state, and national government agencies; professional groups; families; advocacy organizations; academic institutions; and MCH (Maternal and Child Health) policy makers must work together to address the problems of our nation's youth. Coordinated efforts on the part of every organization and at every level will be required. Are there additional measures we should take to reverse these frightening trends? The answer is *yes!* To be effective, they must begin early in a child's life, be multidimensional, intensive, and long-term. I propose six "prescriptions":

1. *Universal, early childhood education* will prepare our children to learn and achieve, removing some of the disadvantages that hold them back. At age four, a child knows half as much as he will ever know. Why, then, are we waiting until kindergarten to intervene academically? Given the success of Head Start in improving school performance, there is no excuse for not making such programs available to all children who need them.

2. *Comprehensive health and family life education* should be taught to all children, starting in kindergarten and continuing through high school. Instruction should be appropriate to the child's ability to understand and need to know, but we must not be timid about facing our obligations to even the youngest children. After all, the messages they get from television and videos, older siblings, and even parents, don't respect their ages. Children need to know about nutrition and physiology and the risks of substance

abuse—tobacco use, alcohol consumption, abuse of prescription medications (more than narcotics alone), and experimentation with substances they may be offered by friends or strangers. In the same way they need to be armed with knowledge about human reproductive biology and development. The risks of early and unprotected sexual activity are effectively learned through such programs. We must do all we can to empower our children with useful facts and resources.

3. *Education and support for parents* in nurturing, caring for, and teaching their children. Many of our social problems are worsened by parents' uninformed attitudes toward health and inappropriate behavior toward their children. Instruction, counsel, and peer discussion should be made available. For our future parents, today's children, this can start in the comprehensive health and family life education opportunities mentioned above. For today's parents, accessible programs must be devised which fit their busy lives. Many settings in our communities can be employed, including churches, civic organizations, work sites, and schools.

4. *Efforts to promote and reinforce responsible behavior by young males.* Family planning and sex education has traditionally focused on young females, thus tacitly absolving young males of sexual responsibility. Like young females, many young males have few opportunities other than procreation to prove themselves. Therefore, we must assure that they also have opportunities for growth and self-expression in other arenas of life.

5. *Comprehensive school-based clinics* are needed to provide medical care, including family planning services, to all teens. Such clinics are logical partners in providing comprehensive health and family life education. If children are taught health promotion and primary prevention and health care, there will be even greater demand for the services of school-based clinics. Providing clinics in schools makes them nearly

universally accessible.

6. *Increased opportunities for higher education.* All children who make good grades, exhibit good citizenship and have a low family income should be guaranteed assistance at state-supported colleges. Our society needs educated critical minds, and our children deserve opportunities to develop fully.

What will it take to fill these prescriptions? Planning, information, and, yes, money. But before much can really happen, our personal and community-wide involvement is critical. Involvement will flow from qualities we find in ourselves. They can be represented by the word **CARE;**

C should remind us of *commitment* to ourselves and our children. This might also be called pride, but it is not shallow.

It is grounded in family love and civic responsibility, the basis of our grandest hopes and most impressive accomplishments.

A represents *awareness* of our world, its needs, and its assets. Combined with intelligence and empathy, awareness can powerfully motivate us to take action.

R is for *responsibility*. Mentally healthy and emotionally secure persons want to help others. They rise to difficult challenges requiring intelligence and sensitivity.

E challenges us to *equip, empower, and encourage* our children—three important duties of all who care for young people. We must fulfill these duties with zeal and skill, drawing on the best in ourselves to secure the promise of a better tomorrow for our children.

If we want to sustain and enhance the quality of life in our nation, we had better move now to save the future. And the future is our children. More than a hundred years ago Abraham Lincoln vividly described our current challenge:

"A child is a person who is going to carry on what you have started. He is going to sit where you are sitting, and when you are gone, attend to those things which you think are important. You may adopt all the policies you please, but how they are carried out depends on him. He will assume control of your cities, states, and nations. He is going to move in and take over your churches, schools, universities and corportations....The fate of humanity is in his hands."

Can We Make a Difference?

The answer is *Yes!* if we:

• ensure early childhood education for all Americans;

• promote widespread health and family life education;

• offer support for all parents in nurturing their children;

• foster responsible behavior by our young men;

• establish a nationwide emphasis on providing school-based clinics;

• make it possible for more young people to benefit from higher education. And if we encourage our society to exercise CARE —a *commitment* to secure a future filled with promise; *awareness* of the needs of all of our citizens; taking *responsibility* to care for our neighbors; working to *equip, empower, and encourage* our children.

14

FOUR

On Poverty and Inequality
Why Don't We Do Something?

For many years we have been living in a throwaway society.

But think about it. How many of us today actively recycle newspapers, glass bottles, aluminum cans, white office paper? Probably none of us was recycling five years ago. The Green Earth movement has done an excellent job educating us about solid-waste landfills that are rapidly filling up with non-biodegradable, disposable diapers and about the threat of the hole in the ozone layer. If you ask any eighth grader today what he or she is worried about, the answer will be, "The environment." Manufactures are picking up on this and rethinking the elaborate packaging of everyday products.

But somehow we still have a disposable, throwaway attitude about our most valuable resource. I mean our children. And when it come to which children are at the greatest disadvantage in today's society, we all know that minority children are still being pushed to the back of the health care bus.

Consider with me the following:

Compared to a white child, a black child is:
- almost three times more likely to be born into poverty;
- twice as likely to be born to a teenage mother;
- twice as likely to be born to a mother who had no prenatal care;
- three times as likely to be born it a dangerously low birth

15

weight (less than 3 pounds, 5 ounces);
- two times more likely to die in the first year of life.

Compared to a white child, a black child has
- a 40 percent greater chance of being born to a mother who did not complete high school;
- three times the chance of being in an educable mentally retarded class;
- less than half the chance of being in a gifted and talented class;
- two and a half times the chance of being suspended from school:

Compared to a white child, a black child is
- three times as likely to be living with only his or her mother;
- four times as likely to be living with neither parent.

Compared to
- a white infant, a black infant is seven times as likely to die of HIV infection;
- her white age peer, a black female age 15 to 24 is five times as likely to die of HIV infection;
- his white age peer, a black male age 15 to 24 is three times as likely to die of HIV infection;
- his or her white age peer, a black child age 1 to 4 is three times as likely to die by firearms;
- his white age peer, a black male age 15 to 19 is almost four times as likely to die by firearms;
- his white age peer, a black male age 20 to 24 is four times as likely to die by firearms.

America is the world's wealthiest nation. But our poorest Americans are the 12 million children who live in poverty. They are the members of what I call the 5-H Club:

> the hungry,
> the homeless,
> the helpless,
> the hugless,
> the hopeless,

The children, who embody our hope for the future, are hanging by a very slender thread to any hope for their own future. Until we address the problems in our society which have resulted in children being poorly housed or homeless, poorly fed, poorly educated, and lacking adequate health care, we will be continuing to hand out bandages when what the patient needs is major surgery.

Everywhere we look, the statistics paint a dismal picture of how our children are doing. Each day

942 infants are born into poverty;

1,334 teenagers become sexually active;

827 teenagers become pregnant;

448 infants are born to teenage mothers;

548 infants are born to mothers who did not graduate from high school;

220 infants are born to mothers who received late or no prenatal care;

56 infants are born with a dangerously low birth weight;

34 infants die;

4 children die by firearms;

5 children are murdered;

6 young adults, age 20 to 24, are murdered;

125 children are arrested for violent crimes;

86 children are arrested for drug crimes;

21 children are arrested for alcohol-related crimes;

544 students drop out of school;

3,374 are suspended from public school.

In the wealthiest nation on earth, we will "trash" nearly 40,000 children this year who will die before their first birthday. Approximately 12,500 of these will be black infants. According to a 1989 White House Task Force Report, at least 25 percent of such deaths could be prevented. It may come as a surprise to note that a black baby born in the United States is less likely to survive than a baby born in Cuba, Jamaica, Trinidad, or Tobago.

One third of our infants and toddlers will go without adequate childhood immunizations. The incidence of preventable communicable diseases has soared. The consequence is that our children are dying. Millions of children are without basic health insurance and access to health care.

Poverty in America

Poverty rates among young families have almost doubled since the mid-1960s, and middle-income families report greater difficulty making ends meet.

Although most poor children are white, minority children are more likely to be poor. Nearly 50 percent of all African-American children and over one-third of Hispanic children live in poverty. The number of black children living in poverty increased by 717,000 between 1979 and 1990 as a result of falling earning among black parents, the declining effectiveness of government aid in lifting children out of poverty, and the increasing proportion of black children living in female-headed families.

Families on average have less income with which to bring up their children. Growth in real wages virtually halted in 1973, and families today spend a higher proportion of their incomes on housing, transportation, health care, higher education and taxes.

Young black men earn far less now than they did in the early 1970s. The average annual earnings of black males ages 20 through 29, after increasing substantially during the 1960s, dropped by one-fourth between 1973 and 1989. Faced with high unemployment and falling wages, increasing proportions of black men have dropped out of the labor force altogether. In 1973, 73 percent of all black men were either employed or looking for work. By 1990, that proportion had dropped to 70 percent.

Contrary to common belief, in most poor families the father is present. However, the chance of being poor increases when there is only one parent. Rising divorce rates and births to single women of all ages have dramatically increased the number and proportion of children being raised in one-parent families. Almost 13 million children live in a single-parent family — almost double the number 20 years ago. We know that a large portion of the 12 million children of the 5-H Club are living in single-parent homes. Minority children are more likely than white children to live in one-parent families. More than half of all African-American children, nearly one-third of all Hispanic children, and almost one-fifth of all white children live today in single-parent families.

In response to the increased difficulties of supporting a

family on one wage, mothers in two-parent families have moved steadily into the work force. In 1970, only 39 percent of families with children had mothers in the work force, but by 1990 that proportion had risen to 61 percent. American families today have less time to devote to the supervision, education, and nurturing of their children than they did two decades ago. The "Ozzie and Harriet family," which was the norm less than thirty years ago, has now become the exception.

Although the federal government recommends that families spend no more than 30 percent of their income for housing, 39 percent of poor black households spend more than half of their incomes for housing. Because this leaves them with very little for other needs, many black families share housing.   In 1990, over 1.8 million black children lived "doubled up," sharing their housing with friends or family. Such arrangements are often a temporary stop between stable housing and homelessness. These families are at high risk of homelessness. According to a 1990 report by the U.S. Conference of Mayors, black people constitute almost half of the homeless population in the nation's cities.

Black educational progress continues to lag behind that of white students. Even though the achievement gap is narrowing, it is still significant. Although black students are finishing high school at a higher rate than in the past, they are still twice as likely to drop out of school as white students. Since 1967, the college-going rate for young black students has increased from 24 percent to 31 percent. However, the college-going rate for white students is now 39 percent.

America's Future

If any of us thinks this is not our problem, let me remind you that our failure to prevent poverty and to address the economic needs of families has led to the social ills we know so well—more crime and delinquency, more teenage childbearing, more unhealthy babies, higher dropout rates, more substance abuse and mental illness, more child abuse and neglect, and lower productivity among the working-age population. These problems are costly, in terms of tax expenditures as well as in human terms. To salvage this disposable population requires significant investments in treatment of chronic health conditions and disabilities, special education, foster care, and welfare. For those we cannot salvage, we have a human landfill called *prison*, and our prisons are being filled beyond capacity at an alarming rate.

If I haven't captured your attention yet, let me explain another reason why we must stop fighting poverty with bandages. Since 1960, the proportion of children in the U.S. population has declined dramatically. In little more than a decade, the labor force will begin to shrink. Although children made up over one-third of the population in 1970, in 1990 they constituted only about one-fourth. The aging of America reflects the convergence of three trends. First, individual Americans are having fewer children than their parents did. Second, baby boomers, those born between 1946 and 1964, are now heading into middle age and out of the primary childbearing years. And, third, more older Americans are living longer. In the foreseeable future, a declining number of workers will have to support a growing number of retirees, you and me!

In the face of an aging population more than ever we need our children to he healthy, skilled, confident, and caring. Today's children are tomorrow's parents, workers, and leaders. The baby born this year will be entering the work force just as the first baby boomers near retirement. While they may not be adequately represented in the current political process, these children will pay the taxes and guide our communities and nation in the early twenty-first century. I plan on being around then, don't you?

Some Lessons

As a leader, each of us shoulders tremendous responsibility. We must draw upon our life experiences to do what we know will make a positive difference. We must remember the lessons of our generation. My friend, and another advocate for children, Marian Wright Edelman, president of the Children's Defense Fund, has synthesized her experiences and submitted "Ten Lessons to Help Us Through the 1990s." They bear repeating.

Lesson 1: There is no free lunch, We must not feel entitled to anything we don't sweat and struggle for. Each of us may take the initiative to create opportunity. A people unable or unwilling to share, to juggle difficult, competing demands, or to make hard choices and sacrifices may be incapable of taking courageous action to rebuild our families and communities and to prepare for the future.

Lesson 2: Set goals and work quietly and systematically toward them. We must resist quick-fix, simplistic answers. We must not talk big and act small. We can't get bogged down in our ego needs. You can achieve a lot if you don't mind working hard and giving others the credit.

Lesson 3: Assign yourself. Don't wait around for your boss or your friends to direct you to do what you are capable of figuring out and doing yourself. Don't do as little as you can to get by. If you see a need, don't ask, "Why doesn't somebody do something?" Ask, "Why don't I do something?"

Lesson 4: Never work just for money. Don't confuse

wealth or fame with character. Don't confuse legality with morality. Refuse to tolerate corruption. And demand that those who represent you do the same.

Lesson 5: Don't be afraid of taking risks or being criticized. An anonymous sage said, "If you don't want to be criticized, don't say anything, do anything, or be anything." It doesn't matter how many times you fall down, it's how many times you get up.

Lesson 6: Take parenting and family life seriously. Our leaders mouth family values that we do not practice. Seventy nations provide medical care and financial assistance to all pregnant women; we are not one of them. Seventeen industrialized nations have paid maternity leave programs; we are not one of them.

Lesson 7: Remember, and help America remember, that the fellowship of human beings is more important than the fellowship of race and class and gender in a democratic society. We must realize that our country's ability to compete and lead in the new century is an inextricably intertwined with our poor and nonwhite children as with white, privileged ones.

Lesson 8: Don't confuse style with substance, or political charm with decency or sound policy. Words alone will not meet our children's or our nation's needs. Leadership and different priorities will.

Lesson 9: Listen for the sound of the genuine within yourself. There are so many competing demands in our lives that many of us never learn to be quiet long enough to hear the sound of the genuine within ourselves or other people.

Lesson 10: Never think that life is not worth living or that you cannot make a difference. In other words, never give up, I know how discouraging it can be to struggle year after year with the same issues. But we have to realize that it isn't necessary to "win" immediately in order to make a difference.

Sojourner Truth, an illiterate slave woman who hated slavery and the second-class treatment of women, was heckled one day by an old white man. "Old woman, do you think that your talk about slavery does any good? Why, I don't care any more for your talk than I do for the bite of a flea."

"Perhaps not," Sojourner rejoined, "but the Lord willing, I'll keep you scratching." Enough committed fleas can make even the biggest dog uncomfortable and transform even the biggest nation.

America can no longer afford to spend more per capita than any other country on personal health care, yet have 37 million citizens within her borders who have little or no health coverage. Every hour, we as a nation spend 33.7 million dollars on our national defense. Yet, we only spend 1.3 million dollars on our children's health.

Unlike murder or suicide, poverty is always a slow death. In behalf of the 12 million children in America who are suffering this fate, I challenge you to get involved, Time is of the essence.

To enlarge on a statement of Statius: A society grows great when old men plant trees under whose shade they know they'll never sit.

Why Don't We Do Something?

How do we move from a society that treats its most valuable resource as non-biodegradable, disposable trash to one in which every child is truly viewed as the most precious gift from God? We must take responsibility for building a hope-filled future. To do so will require that we learn important lessons:

- We must not feel entitled to anything we don't sweat and struggle for.

- We must resist simplistic answers.

- When we are tempted to ask, "Why doesn't somebody do something? We must instead ask, "Why don't I do something?"

- We must keep our priorities straight, act honestly, and expect others to do the same.

- We must be willing to take risks.

- We must take our roles as members of families seriously.

- We must remember that the future lies with all children.

- We must demand leadership and never be satisfied with words alone.

- We must never, ever give up.

Notes

Center for the Study of Social Policy, *Kids County Data Book*, WashingtonD.C.,1991.
Children's Defense Fund. *State of America's Children 1991*, Washington, D.C. 1991.
Children's Defense Fund. *Health of America's Children*. Washington, D.C., 1992.
Gans, Janet E., Ph. D. *America's Adolescents: How Healthy Are They?* Chicago: American Medical Association, 1990.
LaBella, Arleen, and Dolores Leach. Personal Power. Boulder, Colo. 1983.
National Commission on the Role of the School and the Community in Improving Adolescent Health. *Code Blue: Uniting for Healthier Youth*. Alexandria, VA., 1990

National Commission on Children. *Beyond Rhetoric: A New American Agenda for Children and Families.* Washington, D.C., 1991

Randall-Davis, Elizabeth, Ph.D. *Strategies for Working with Culturally Diverse Communities and Clients.* Washington, D. C.: Association for the Care of Children, 1989.

Shames, Steven and Jonathan Kozol. *Outside the Dream: Child Poverty in America.* Washington, D.C.: Children's Defense Fund, 1991.

FIVE

On School Health Services
How Do We Get Started

Schools of the twenty-first century will be the centerpiece of communities. They will provide not only the three R's, but will serve as the hub for the integration of health, mental health, social, and support services for children and families.

Economic and social factors have seriously eroded the integrity and functioning of the American family, contributing to a wide range of social problems involving, children and youth even prior to their beginning school. These problems include not only poor social and academic development, but also poor physical and mental health; abuse of drugs and alcohol and their related conditions; exposure to domestic and community violence and abuse; teenage pregnancy and the need to assume parental responsibilities prematurely; limited employment preparation, opportunities, and role models; and family disorganization and dysfunction.

If we expect all children to reach their educational potential, then we must equip schools to address these multifaceted problems as they are presented. In recent years, the relationship between good health and learning has received growing attention in many areas of the nation. To improve the accessibility of health services, many schools are placing health care providers in the public schools where children spend most of their time.

School-based health services are convenient for students,

parents, and teachers; they are cost effective for payors, confidential for the student, and provide comprehensive integration of services for the student and family that are age appropriate.

The following describes the success of school-based health clinics in the state of Arkansas, where I served as director of the Department of Health. By ensuring that consensus is reached by all interested parties—school boards, local health units, and community leaders during clinic development, implementation, and evaluation—Arkansas has been able to show that the health care needs of many children can effectively and efficiently be met through a school-based program of health services. Some of the planning steps required prior to the establishment of school health services are shown in Table I. Questions to be addressed by the school, involved agencies, and the community are shown in Table II. The role of school leadership is summarized in Table III. The process of designing a school health program and the components of a comprehensive school health program are shown in Tables IV and V. Table VI lists criteria for effective school-based or school-linked health services, while Table VII contains a resolution addressing the issue of teenage pregnancy in Arkansas.

Defining School Health Services

A critical key to development of a clinic is understanding and agreeing on the types of health services that can be delivered at school. *The Journal of School Health* (1987, page 411) defines school-based health services as follow:

School health service programs promote the health of students through prevention, case finding, early intervention, and remediation of specific health problems, provision of first aid and triage of illness and

28

injuries, provision of direct services for handicapped students, and provision of health counseling and health instruction for faculty, staff and students. Professionally-prepared school nurses most often coordinate and provide the health services program. However, there are other professionals who provide specific services to promote the health and well-being of the school-age child, including school physicians, dentists, social workers, and speech pathologists.

The Arkansas Department of Health has broadened this definition to embrace the following philosophy:

School-based health services provide accessible, affordable and preventive health services in the schools. The goal of school-based health services is to improve the overall physical and emotional health of children and adolescents. This is accomplished by providing good quality, accessible health care to children when they need it. School-based health services also promote healthy life-styles so youth will have less need for health care. This is accomplished by enriching classroom experiences to include teaching about preventive health care and consumer behaviors and promoting the development of good decision-making skills in relation to health and other life issues.

Each school district should define school-based health services according to the needs of the children and the concerns of its community. A small but vocal portion of some communities has the misperception that school-based health services are "sex clinics" which provide only reproductive health care or abortion referral services. In reality, data indicate that only 15 percent of clinic visits concern reproductive health, and many of these visits are associated with treatment of sexually transmitted diseases.

Developing a School District, Health Department and Community Partnership

The Arkansas Department of Health received funds from several sources to develop, implement, and evaluate school-based health services. In order to effectively allocate the money to schools, each school district in Arkansas was polled to ascertain its interest in providing school-based health services. Those school districts choosing to participate provided documentation of the need for, and their willingness to support, school-based health services.

It was incumbent on school districts to provide evidence of support for school-based health services by developing and submitting a proposal along with a letter of support from the school's superintendent. Because the superintendent is hired by the school board, whose members are elected from the community, a letter from the superintendent was assumed to imply community support.

To ensure program funding and success, each proposal had to address the following areas:

- formation of a planning group to determine health needs and to set goals for the school-based health services program;
- evidence of parental and community-based support and approval for school-based health services; and
- formulation of a plan to provide an information campaign to parents and community about school-based health services. In order to receive favorable review, the school superintendent, local health unit, and community leaders all had to be involved in proposal development.

Specifying the Role and Responsibility
of School Leadership

If school-based or school-linked services are to be adequately implemented, there must be a significant commitment to participate by all levels of school personnel, district leadership, middle management, principals, and teachers. The district superintendent and local board of trustees can initiate the planning process, or it can be initiated in conjunction with the local health or social service agency.

Regardless of who initiates the service, the school superintendent and governing body of the school district must be involved from the beginning and must view themselves as equals with other community agency executives involved in the process. School staff and school principals need the commitment and involvement of district leadership to pave the way for meaningful restructuring and delivery of integrated school health services.

School district leaders with executives from other agencies must undertake two essential tasks in planning for school-based services. First, a needs assessment must be conducted to clarify various factors at work in the community, its demographics, racial composition, cultural and language diversity, poverty levels, and other indicators of risk for students. Next, a mission statement should be drafted to delineate the purpose of collaboration in establishing clinics, the children and families to be served, the scope of services, the expected outcomes, and the funding sources. The answers to these questions must be tailored to the strengths and needs of each community and the participating agencies.

School superintendents, board members, and other

agency executives cannot implement school-based services without the involvement of mid-level managers. Middle managers serve as the important link between a change in policy at the executive level and an actual change in action below. They serve as liaisons with the principals and teachers of the district and as the line staff of other agencies.

The school principal must be willing to assume new roles and utilize new skills to successfully implement a school-based service effort. It is likely that prior leadership training for the principal did not emphasize collaborative leadership and shared decision-making with outside community agencies. These skills, however, are essential.

First, the principal must be an active participant in developing the services that are to be associated with the school. The principal's chief tasks include sharing information about the children and community, connecting the planning group to parents and teachers, and providing a reality check for planners who may not understand the day-to-day functions of the school. The principal also maintains chief responsibility for the school clinic, as for any other service in his or her school.

Second, the principal must act as a school-based clinic advocate, working with families and other agencies, stating the case to his or her peers, the community, and the school staff.

Third, the principal must recognize and link key teachers and other school staff with persons from the community health and social service agencies in order to assure that optimal services are provided for his or her patients or clients, the students.

Fourth, the principal must act as an enabler, promoting the involvement of other staff and community members in planning and monitoring a school-linked service effort. Success of such services depends on the active involvement of teachers at the school site, both as teaching and support staff for the clinic.

Evaluating School-based Health Services to Reflect Successes, Progress and Community Support

Since the first school-based health services were established in Arkansas' public schools, program success has been documented by the majority of schools through their impact on health-related problems such as a decreased incidence of teenage pregnancy, substance abuse, sexually transmitted diseases, injuries, homicides, and suicides. In addition, schools with successful school based health services have demonstrated a decrease in the number of dropouts, an increased awareness among staff, teachers, parents, and students about health-related problems, and a reduction of risk-taking behaviors among students.

An Example of School-linked Services

The Arkansas Department of Health established uniform data collection methods in school-based clinics in order to evaluate the quantity and quality of services offered through the program. Such data will provide feedback to the clinic staff, the school district, and the community, as well as serve as the basis for seeking additional funding to expand school-based services to other schools.

Although school-based health services were established with only teenage pregnancy reduction in mind at first, the clinic's services have gradually evolved into an array of health services seeking to improve the overall health of the student body. Some of the health-related services currently offered at the clinic are follow-up exams, WIC (a supplmental nutrition program for women, infants, and children), blood pressure screening, and immunizations. In addition, school-based health services have been established in conjunction and a summer recreational program for school-age children.

Leon A. Phillips, Jr., Superintendent of Schools in the Lakeview School District in eastern Arkansas, believes there are several issues that should be addressed when planning for school-based health services. First, consult the community and local school board about establishing school-based health services. Educate the community as to why a school-based clinic is needed. Assemble a community group to provide guidance in the selection of clinic services and clinic operation. The school district board of trustees should approve the clinic.

It is also important to develop and maintain good public relations with churches and other community groups. A positive attitude toward school-based health services is critical. And easy access to the clinic should be established. The clinic must be located on the site for students to easily avail themselves of services while in school. Written parental consent for students to utilize clinic services should be obtained at the beginning of each school year, or when a student is enrolled. Arkansas utilizes a checklist that allows parents to specify what services, if any, they do not want their children to receive.

Barriers or Roadblocks

The most common roadblocks or barriers encountered

have been: (a) lack of knowledge by the general public of the health problems of students; (b) misconceptions or myths of what goes on in a school-based clinic; (c) religious leaders who have concerns as to whose values will be taught and if children are taught about human sexuality they will "do it"; (d) failure to get the community involved in the project and have them adopt it as their idea; (e) errors in staffing; and (f) the cost of providing school-based clinic services. The average cost of school-based clinic services in Arkansas has been approximately $100 per child. The average cost of health insurance in America today, however, is greater than $2,500 per person and does not provide preventive health care, which is the single greatest need of children.

How Do We Get Started?

When deciding whether school-based health services are needed in a school or school district, the superintendent and other administrative personnel need to determine the following:

- What health-related information about student populations is easily accessible (e.g., vital statistics, youth risk factor behavior survey)?

- What will be the school district's working definition or philosophy of school-based health services?

- What school-based health services are needed and why?

- What partnerships need to be formed with key community groups to provide consultation and support for school-based health services?

■ How can community-based planning be approached which will be inclusive of and responsive to the children's needs?

Answering these questions will give the school district a strong foundation upon which to build a school-based health services?

TABLE I

Planning Steps Required Prior to Establishment of School Health Services

—A planning group from the local community must be formed to determine health needs and set goals for the school health service program.

—A site must be selected to enable planning to center around activities for the locale.

—Community-based support and approval must be obtained in order to begin a comprehensive program.

—An information campaign should be utilized to provide clear, concise answers to the community's questions about the program.

—Demonstrated support of school officials and parents is crucial to the establishment of a comprehensive school health service program.

TABLE II

Questions to Ask in Designing a School-based or School-linked Service Strategy

—What is the primary purpose or objective of the strategy?

—Who is to be served?

—What services will be offered?

—Where will services be located?

—Who will be responsible for service delivery?

TABLE III

The Role of School Leadership in Developing School-based Health Services

—Develop an understanding of the role, function, and services of school-based clinics.
—Serve as a liaison with school board.
—Organize town meetings to inform the community.
—Serve as a liaison with media.
—Serve as a liaison with parents.
—Assess the needs of students.
—Communicate these needs to the community.
—Enlist the support of churches and other organizations.
—Enlist the support of parents.
—Make clinic space and support personnel available.

TABLE IV

Designing a School Health Program

—Parental consent must be obtained in order to provide care to children.
—A consolidated, wholistic approach to the health care needs of the children must be evident.
—A variety of services would be available to prevent fragmentation of care and to promote student use of the service.

- A caring, youth-oriented staff must be available to provide care and establish rapport with students and the community.
- Each patient must be given the opportunity to spend ample time with caregivers to promote trust and to allow for adequate assessment of patient needs.
- A detailed follow-up procedure for referrals and missed appointments must be developed.
- Cooperative relationships with other community providers and agencies must be developed and maintained by the clinic staff.
- Data on visit, compliance rates, and illnesses treated must be collected for program monitoring and evaluation.

TABLE V

Components of a Comprehensive School Health Program
Health Assessments/Physical Examinations

- Routine screening physicals (scoliosis, hearing/speech/vision where applicable-sports physicals
- Gynecological exams/cancer screening
- EPSDT screening (Early Periodic Screening, Diagnosis, and Treatment)
- Blood pressure screening
- Dental Screening
- Screening for infants of adolescents (if in school / day care)
- Immunization status
- WIC assessment (Women, Infants, and Children)

Assessment and Referral of Minor Illness, Disease, and Injury

- Flu and colds

- Earaches (otitis media)
- Sprains, cuts, burns
- Sore throats (e.g., strep)
- Dermatologic conditions (acne, dermatitis, impetigo)
- Minor gynecological problems (vaginitis, yeast)
- Menstrual disorders / dysmenorrhea
- Sexually transmitted diseases
- Urinary tract infections-acute
- Anemia

Counseling/Education

- Abstinence / sexuality education (menstruation)
- Contraceptive methods (referrals, prescriptions, dispensing)
- Sexually transmitted disease counseling
- Nutrition/weight reduction/weight management
- Smoking prevention and cessation
- Stress management
- Alcohol and drug abuse prevention
- Safety (seat belts, car seats, helmets)
- Parenting classes
- Suicide prevention
- Family counseling
- Mental health and psychosocial counseling
- Job counseling and employment training
- Pegnancy counseling
- Breast self-exam
- Testicular self-exam
- WIC counseling if applicable
- Abuse counseling

Home Visitation

For at-home counseling with parents, students, follow-up of problems:

Referrals for Follow-up for Major Health Problems

— Chronic diseases (e.g.,diabetes, hypertension)

— Eating disorders (anorexia/bulimia)

— Alcohol and drug abuse

— Suicide prevention counseling

— High-risk prenatal patients/problems and delivery services

— Major gynecological problems

— Other surgical problems (tumors, etc.)

— Infectious disease epidemics

Sanitation Services
— Environmental health

— School safety inspections

— Asbestos testing

Laboratory Testing as Appropriate

— Hematocrit/hemoglobin

— VDRL

— Gonorrhea culture

— Pap smear

— Pregnancy test

- PKU
- Urinalysis
- Weight
- Height
- Blood pressure

Table VI

Criteria for Effective School-based or School-linked Health Services

- Participating agencies will need to change how they deliver services to children and families and how they work together.

- Planning and implementation cannot be dominated by any one institution—school, health, or social service agency.

- Services need to be comprehensive and tailored to the needs of individual children and families.

- Each agency participating should redirect some of its current funding to support the new collaboration.

- Services should involve and support parents and the family as a whole.

- Schools must be willing to collect and evaluate data.

- Schools must respond to the diversity of children and families. Modified from the *Future of Children*, volume 2, number 1 (Spring 1992) School Linked Services. The David and Lucile Pachard Foundation.

TABLE VII

Resolution in the Matter of Teenage Pregnancy in Arkansas

WHEREAS   teenage pregnancy has profound effects on the lives of the adolescent, her unborn child, her male partner, her family, and on society as a whole; and

WHEREAS   teenage pregnancy is associated with numerous socioeconomic and health problems, including but not limited to, low educational achievement, unemployment welfare, pregnancy-related health risks, infant morbidity, mortality and abuse; and

WHEREAS   8,874 teenage women became pregnant in Arkansas in 1986; and

WHEREAS   1,1996 of these pregnancies (22%) were terminated by abortion; and

WHEREAS   6,595 of these pregnancies resulted in live births, which accounted for 19% of all live births in Arkansas; and

WHEREAS   190 of these births were to adolescents under the age of 15; and

WHEREAS   3,502 of these mothers were unwed; and

WHEREAS   the divorce rate for teen women who are married is 2.5 times that of women over the age of 20 when they marry; and

WHEREAS   10,807 women received prenatal care in Arkansas public health clinics in 1986; and

WHEREAS   approximately 31% of these women were 19 years of age or younger, and

42

WHEREAS   throughout this country, where teen health
            centers have provided family planning
            services, including prescriptive capacity,
            the rate of adolescent pregnancy has been
            significantly reduced; and
WHEREAS   the Arkansas State Board of Health has made
            a commitment to the ongoing funding of
            prevention and early intervention programs
            for youth,

NOW THEREFORE BE IT RESOLVED that the
Arkansas State Board of Health creates the following policy
regarding teenage pregnancy:

1. that we do not condone or encourage sexual activity among
   adolescents:
2. that communication with parents regarding all health care
   matters will be encouraged;
3. that sexually active teenagers may receive counselling on
   responsible family planning and health services in
   keeping with Arkansas State Law (Act 235 of 1973);
4. that at the invitation of individual communities and with
   the approval of the local school board, school-based
   counseling and clinic services may be initiated;
5. that when a sexually active adolescent does become
   pregnant, appropriate prenatal care, counseling, and
   supportive referrals may be given;
6. that when a pregnant adolescent does deliver a baby,
   appropriate agencies may be contacted to assist with
   adoption or teen parenting skill-building, counseling,
   education, and referrals;
7. that the goal of this policy of the Arkansas State Board of
   Health is to reduce the incidence of teenage pregnancy
   and its devastating effects on the lives of our citizens.

This document has been styled after a resolution of the Board of County Commis-
sioners, Multnomah County, Oregon, as printed in *Healthy Children*, a publication and
program administered by Harvard University's Division of Health Policy Research and Education. Healthy Children is supported by a grant from the Robert Wood Johnson Foundation.

SIX

On Learning and Self-esteem
How Do We Motivate for Change?

The second decade of life is a time of rapid physical growth and development. Most of us remember our adolescence as a challenging and confusing time—a time when energy levels were high, appetites strong, and our bodies blossomed into adulthood.

But young people today face a very different adolescence. For the first time in the history of this country, young people are less healthy and less prepared to take their places in society than were their parents.

These facts are often quoted but deserve repeating:

In 1950, a group of sociologists conducted a survey. Many of us can resonate with its finding. The major problems in our school system were these:

1. Talking in class
2. Chewing gum
3. Being disruptive in class
4. Running through the halls
5. Getting out of line when asked to line up
6. Wearing improper clothes
7. Failing to put paper in baskets

Recently the same group of sociologists did another survey. The most pressing problems in our schools today are these:

1. Drug abuse
2. Alcohol abuse

3 Pregnancy
4. Suicide
5. Rape
6. Robbery
7. Assault

- Every seven seconds a student drops out of school.

- Every 67 seconds a teenagers has a baby

- Every seven minutes a child is arrested for drugs.

- Every year 700,000 children receive a high school diploma that they cannot read.

- America ranks fourteenth out of fifteen industrialized countries tested in math. Hong Kong was first, and Japan was second.

- America ranks thirteenth out of fifteen tested in science, ninth out of ten in chemistry, and seventh out of ten in physics.

- The Centers for Disease control in Atlanta estimates that each year 2.5 million adolescents contract a sexually transmitted disease.

- Every day 135,000 American students bring guns to school.

- The homicide rate has doubled among 10- to 14-year olds during the past twenty years and is the leading cause of death among black 15- to 19-year-olds during the past twenty years.

The compelling problems of our young people are

readily indentifiable. However, the causes are more complicated to define. The problems facing children during puberty and adolescence are not uniquely associated with the physical changes their bodies are experiencing. Children today face a different America. Deep-rooted changes have occurred in our society over the last two decades and have drastically affected our children. Our society is more complex, more challenging, and more competitive than ever before. Changes in our families and our neighborhoods have robbed our youth of necessary guidance and support. Americans are more mobile, poverty is increasing, more families require a second income, and our lives are faster paced.

These children, on whom we will depend for decisions in the twenty-first century, face problems that threaten their ability to become healthy adults capable of leading full, productive lives. Business leaders and educators agree that the labor force of the future will need educated, healthy adults if the United States is to remain competitive in the global economy. Adolescents who are sick, hungry, or abused, who are distracted by family problems, who drink or use drugs, and who feel they have no chance to succeed in the world are unlikely to attain the level of education required for success in the twenty-first century. Many will be marginally employable, threatening our nation's productivity and competitiveness.

I have outlined in Chapter 3 six prescriptions to address the diseases that plague us. To implement needed changes, we must motivate all people in communities to take part in making a positive difference. How do we do that? All adults must provide committed and competent leadership.

There are many persons in every sector of our nation

who have the necessary skills and who have demonstrated courage and tenacity in providing such leadership. But all of us must work harder. Some will argue that there are no leaders, others say that we have too few leaders, a few claim that there are enough leaders, or that there are too many leaders of the wrong sort.

We most often see leadership as a personal quality, something that a person has intrinsically as part of his or her personality, a quality that makes him or her stand out. We say that someone is a born leader, a natural leader, or that he or she has innate leadership qualities and abilities.

It is often hard to imagine ourselves as leaders. We often view leaders as "super-people," able to keep going seemingly without limits of time or energy. Thus, people who lead ordinary lives, with a job (or two or three), kids, aging parents, mortgages, plumbing that leaks, and a car that breaks down may be discouraged from ever trying to be leaders. But I say, broaden your vision; become a leader. Let's consider more fully the word *leader* and what it means:

The *l* in *leader* is for *learn*. You must learn what the needs and problems are in your own community. You must identify all available allies: schools, churches, hospitals, service agencies, key businesses, community and political leaders. You must also learn who may present obstacles; learning includes getting to know the opposition. Then identify someone who can help you bridge the gap. Often, leadership means finding and encouraging key persons who will stand up and support us at critical times.

The *e* is for *educate*. There are those who feel the programs I want for children are morally wrong. I believe it's morally wrong for children to go hungry, it's morally wrong for children to be cold, and it's morally wrong for children to be poor. If we had a perfect society, with no hungry children and a place for everyone to live, there would be no need for the programs I advocate. I often ask people if they are willing to let a baby die of hunger just because his mother did something wrong. Once educated, the majority of people support needed programs.

The *a* in *leader* is for *advocacy*. Sometimes we get so busy arguing, working, and planning for our own particular programs that we forget we are a part of a larger and interrelated system. It takes the efforts of many people to make effective and needed programs work; it takes the schools, the mothers, the fathers, the churches—everybody in the community. We must attract diverse groups in order to build a viable infrastructure for our programs. Each agency or group must work with others, playing its own role. Over and over again, superior programs without adequate infrastructures have simply disappeared with the departure of their founders.

The *d* in *leader* is for *design*. We have to design and develop programs that are unique and fit the special needs of individual communities. This is illustrated by an old Chinese fable. A monkey and a fish were caught in a great flood. The agile monkey was able to scramble up a tree to safety. Looking down into the raging waters, he saw a fish struggling against the swift current. Filled with a desire to help his less fortunate fellow, he reached down and scooped the fish from the water. To the monkey's surprise, the fish was not very grateful for his aid.

Many communities have a long history of outsiders coming in to "rescue" their members from some inherent danger. Although well meaning, many of these programs are ineffective because they do not involve community members in the planning and implementation.

The second *e* in *leader* is for *enable*. Communities do not want to be told by outsiders what their problems are and how to solve them. In the spirit of community pride and self-determination, they want assistance to enable them to help themselves. Local leaders have a right to expect the "experts" to offer assessment and assistance, but unless the local community assumes responsibility for making something happen in their hometowns, the efforts will be to no avail. We must enable people to overcome their problems.

Finally, the *r* in *leader* is for *responsibility* and *risk-taking*. It is our responsibility to reach out, and that often means taking risks. We may see risk as inevitably ending in ruin, injury, hurt, and loss and, therefore, as something to avoid. We should, however, think of a mistake as an occasional misstep on our path toward our goal. Viewed in this light, mistakes can even be positive. They are an important aspect of self-education; there is almost always a valuable lesson to be learned from failure. A perfect record is not a statement of invincibility, but more likely an indication that we simply are not taking enough risks.

When people say they are daunted by the challenge of becoming leaders, I draw upon my person experience to encourage them to do their part in building a hope-filled future for our children. I have learned that there is nothing mystical about being a leader. To begin with, it's hard work. Second, leaders take a lot of flak. Being a leader is sometimes an isolating experience. But Americans have a heritage of compassion and conscientiousness, and I believe our efforts are needed now more than ever before. If we want to keep our nation as we know it, we had better move to save the future—and the future is our children.

How Do We Motivate for Change?

We become leaders willing to take risks to make a positive difference by:

- learning about the needs and problems in our communities and identifying available resources to address them;
- educating others so that the base of support and involvement will grow ever larger;
- advocating for the involvement of diverse groups in building the needed infrastructure for effective programs;
- designing solutions that are unique and fit the special needs of individual communities;
- enabling persons to find the resources and support to help themselves;
- taking responsibility.

SEVEN

On a Healthy America
How Can We Increase Access to
Health Care Services?

America currently faces one of her most critical domestic policy agendas ever. Reform of the nation's health care system simultaneously presents a staggering challenge and an exciting opportunity. The health of our nation is inextricably entwined with the health of our citizens. In order to meet the multifaceted challenges of the twenty-first century, we must have a healthy America — citizens who are capable of leading socially and economically productive lives.

The current U.S. health care system is not producing a healthy America. Costs are out of control, and many Americans are not receiving needed health care services. The statistics are compelling:

- U.S. health care spending grew from less than 6 percent of the gross national product (GNP) in 1960 to more than 12 percent in 1990. This trend is expected to continue, with the U.S. spending $817 billion, or 14 percent of the GNP, on health care in 1992.

- Overall spending on health care increased by 163 percent from 1980 to 1990, rising from $230 billion to $606 billion.

- During the 1980s' spending for employer-based health insurance premiums increased 164 percent, rising from $66 billion to $174 billion a year.

- Out of pocket spending for individuals increased 157 percent during the 1980s.

- Per capita health care costs in the Unites States are the highest in the world.

Unfortunately, despite the $700 billion the nation spends on health care each year, there have not been corresponding improvements in health status. The health status in the United States is not conspicuously superior to that of other countries, and by some measures it is clearly inferior. Canada, Germany, Great Britain, and Japan spend substantially less on health per capita and as a percentage of GNP, but have lower infant mortality rates for low-risk and moderate-risk surgery, and higher life expectancies for both men and women.

It is important to remember that we are all affected by soaring health care costs. The cost of reform is often debated without reference to what we currently spend. People without health insurance do receive health services, though often less than they need, and on a delayed basis or in an inappropriate setting. Prices of private health insurance are higher to compensate providers for the care they render to the uninsured. Property taxes are higher to support public hospitals serving a disproportionate share of uninsured patients. The lack of preventive and primary care leads many to overuse more expensive services, and inappropriate patterns of health care use create a major drain on health expenditures. Thus, the question for policymakers, providers, and patients is not whether we will pay for health care, but how we choose to pay.

Health insurance coverage and access to health care services are fundamentally linked in the United States

Research conducted over the last decade supports the notion that having or lacking insurance coverage is related to access to services; to the types, quality, and intensity of the care delivered; and to patient health. Uninsured persons are up to three times more likely than privately insured individuals to use health care services at a lower rate, receive potentially inadequate health care, and suffer adverse health outcomes. Individuals with public coverage may be slightly better off than those who are uninsured. Uninsured Americans have been found to be up to 1.3 times more likely than publicly insured individuals to experience a lower health care utilization rate, and 1.5 times more likely than privately insured patients to experience potentially inadequate health services, and up to 4 times more likely to experience an adverse health outcome.

In 1990, an estimated 34.4 million individuals, or 15.7 percent of the population under age 65, were uninsured either all or part of the year. Surprisingly, however, about three-quarters of the uninsured work or are dependents of workers. Half of the uninsured are employed by small businesses.

There are a number of factors that affect an individual's ability to obtain insurance through the workplace. While 81.7 percent of full-time workers have insurance, only 62 percent of part-timers and 54.3 percent of the self-employed are covered. Coverage also varies by industry. Industries in which the work is frequently seasonal, unskilled, or more likely to be non-unionized have much lower rates of employer-provided insurance. But perhaps the most important factor with regard to the workplace that affects the availability of health benefits is business size. Fewer than half the firms with twenty or fewer employees offered health benefits to any of their employees in 1989.

Lack of insurance coverage is particularly dramatic among the young adult population. More than 30 percent of persons between the ages of nineteen and twenty-five are uninsured. This is because often young people were covered as dependents on a parent's policy, and then they face an interim period of job status. Young children must rely on their parents for coverage, and in 1986, 36 percent of the uninsured children were in homes where the family head had health coverage. And, finally, while 12 percent of whites are uninsured, 22 percent of blacks and 32 percent of Hispanics lack insurance coverage, to a certain extent mirroring the workplace situations of these populations.

However, all is not well for those with insurance. Many insurance companies deny coverage to individuals with pre-existing conditions such as cancer, heart disease, diabetes, and asthma. And underinsurance — when coverage is inadequate and the individual or family does not have the means to absorb the required out-of-pocket expenses — has become increasingly common. Employer benefit coverage has eroded as rising costs have caused employers to shift more and more of the health benefit costs to employees. Premium increases, in combination with increasing deductibles and co-insurance that rises in proportion to medical costs, have resulted in out-of-pocket expenditures rising faster than medical care prices in the 1980s. Individuals can face catastrophic costs if their policy places an upper limit on the number of hospital days or a maximum payout of benefits. Most Americans are two paychecks away from medical indigence!

Many insurance packages exclude coverage for pregnancy and primary prevention. Only 42 percent of insurance policies cover immunizations. Children who have private insurance are often referred to public clinics for vaccinations because their insurance does not cover routine immunizations. This has resulted in a decline in the percentage of children fully immunized against childhood diseases, and an increase in preventable diseases such as measles.

Increasing access to health care services is complex. Significant and formidable barriers exist because of geography, availability of health care professionals, ethnic and cultural differences, and, in the case of rural America, the constant threat of closure of hospitals, clinics, and other rural health care providers. Unless such issues as resource development, capacity building, transportation, and outreach are addressed, many Americans will continue to experience significant barriers to accessing essential health care services.

More than 570,000 physicians practice medicine in the United States today—almost double the number twenty years ago. Yet, the proportion practicing primary care has declined. The shortage of general practitioners also leads to further waste of medical resources. Without a family doctor, people are left to find their way through a costly medical system, often seeking high-priced help where the skills of a generalist would have been sufficient.

Rural areas, in particular, face multiple challenges in recruiting and retaining providers: lower expected income, inadequate income to pay overhead, liability insurance, medical loans, limited availability of nearby hospitals, professional isolation, and a lack of amenities for providers and their families compared with metropolitan areas.

But rural communities are not the only underserved areas. Big cities also face shortages of physicians. Physicians are less likely to set up inner-city practices because of limited earnings potential and cultural and language differences.

A sufficient number and an appropriate mix of health care providers must be trained to meet the needs of underserved areas. We must support not only physicians as providers of primary care, but a variety of other providers, including certified nurse midwives, nurse practitioners, physician assistants, and others, in teams and individually, as appropriate. Scholarship and loan programs, tax credits, supplemental payments, and regulation of health care facilities can also be used to improve the availability of services in underserved areas.

The access problem is further driven and compounded by health care costs. Health care inflation continues to rise faster than general inflation. Sophisticated technology to diagnose and treat disease has outstripped society's ability to pay for it. Cost containment is supported by insurance reform and increases emphasis on primary and preventive services, but we must also look for ways to reduce administrative overhead, whether it is in the marketing of insurance, the multiplicity of overlapping utilization, or the complexity of billing and payment procedures. We need strategies to reduce the rate of capital investment in duplicative services, technology, and facilities within defined geographic areas. Malpractice must be addressed through tort reform, alternative dispute resolution, and/or the application of practice guidelines as a defensible standard. Any national health plan would have quality assurance systems and accountability mechanisms that ensure continuous reexamination of and improvement in health care service delivery. There is a real need to systematically provide the public with information about health care. We must ensure that citizens have access to medical care, and that health care services are evaluated against appropriate standards to ensure that the services people receive are effective.

While concern about financial access is legitimate and has been the central focus of the public policy debate, efforts to use our resources more effectively and efficiently must be pursued just as vigorously. High medical expenditures do not consistently translate into improved quality of life or greater life expectancy. Health promotion and disease prevention efforts are the base of the health care system. Scarce health care dollars can be better spent for services that promote and maintain health. The cost-effectiveness of preventive and primary care is well documented: For example:

- Teenage pregnancies cost the government more than $20 a year, yet a $1 investment in family planning services saves more than $4 in health and welfare costs.

- It costs $50,000 on average, before a low-birth-weight baby can leave the hospital, but it costs only $4,800 for comprehensive prenatal and delivery care.

- It costs $15,000 a year to educate a child born addicted to drugs or alcohol, but it only costs $3,000 per year to educate a healthy child. Truly, an ounce of prevention is worth a pound of cure!

Traditional public health programs are the core of preventive activities. Prevention at its most basic level includes health promotion; disease prevention, including screening, early detection, early care and treatment; epidemiologic services; and environmentally safe air, water, and food supplies for the communities. In addition, population-based prevention activities extend beyond the boundaries of individual providers. For example, lead poisoning, vaccine preventable diseases, tuberculosis, and infant mortality require community-wide services, including outreach, screening, linkage to care, monitoring, and education. Recent lapses in the support of basic prevention functions have resulted in new epidemics of communicable diseases that had been controlled.

Preventive and primary services should be community based. Community health care systems must be strengthened and expanded to safeguard health and educate citizens about their capacities to maintain their health. Positive changes in health status are possible if effective preventive and primary services are adopted at the community and provider level. An intensified system for educating and encouraging the American people to change any behavior that results in ill health and high costs should remind persons of their responsibility to maintain their own health. Such programs should be carried out wherever people are—homes, schools, work sites, churches, gyms, and so on. And even with universal health insurance coverage, certain population groups, such as the homeless, persons with AIDS, and drug-addicted babies, will continue to require special consideration in the development and provision of targeted and enhanced health care services.

Reforming the health care system in America is a monumental challenge. Success will require extraordinary will, risk taking, and the development of unlikely coalitions of interested persons. Fear of change must be overcome, for the costs of inaction are unacceptably high. If we can't face the choices now, too many children will continue to come to school unprepared to learn, too many adolescents will continue to face serious but preventable health problems, and too many adults will be prevented from leading full and productive lives. America cannot afford to accept any less than a health care system that provides all citizens with access to appropriate services at affordable prices. Our future depends upon it.

How Can We Increase Access to Health Care Services?

We can begin now to institute major reforms to address pressing problems including the following:

- The current U.S. health care system is not producing a healthy America.

- Too many Americans are not covered by medical insurance; current plans often limit access to health care; and ceilings on benefits could threaten the financial well-being of most Americans.

- Barriers to health care access exist because of geography, availability of health care professionals, ethnic and cultural differences, and in the case of rural America, the constant threat of closure of hospitals and clinics.

- The U.S. faces a shortage of general practitioners over all and in rural areas and the inner cities specifically.

- The rapid rate of health care cost inflation continues to rise faster than general inflation. Sophisticated technologies and overlapping services within communities have led to costs which have outstripped our ability to pay.

- Recent lapses in the support of basic prevention functions have resulted in new epidemics of communicable diseases that have been controlled.

Remember, persons must be willing to make a positive

difference. Fear of change must be overcome, for the costs of inaction are unacceptably high.

Sources

American Public Health Association. *A National Health Program for All of Us.* Washington, D.C.., 1991

Association of State and Territorial Health Officials. *Statement on Health Care Reform.* Washington, D.C. , May, 1992.

Castro, Janice. "Condition: Critical," *Time,* November 25, 1991

Meyer, Jack A.: Sharon Silow-Carroll; and Sean Sullivan. *A National Health Plan in the U.S., The Long-Term Impact on Business and the Economy.* Washington, D.C..: Economic and Social Research Institute, 1991.

National Governors' Association. *A Healthy America: The Challenge for States.* Washington, D.C., 1991.

National Rural Health Association. *National Health Policy Reform: The Rural Perspective.* Kansas City, Mo., September 1992.

Office of Technology Assessment, Congress of the United States. *Does Health Insurance Make a Difference?* Washington, D.C., 1991

EIGHT

On the Role of the Churches
How Can We Help People Who Are Suffering

We all owe the many churches and church organizations in America our thanks for things they do, each and every day. Religious organizations are providing outstanding leadership in areas such as health care and are working to stamp our oppression and hunger. I know that this is so because the church has been very important in shaping my own life.

When I was fifteen years old and graduating from high school, I had never been out of my small community. I received on graduation night the opportunity for a full scholarship to Philander Smith College, if I could get there. At that time, I had never even thought of college. But with the promise of a scholarship in hand, my sisters and brothers picked cotton for me to earn my bus fare to go to Philander Smith College. My little brother, who is now a District Superintendent (regional leader in The United Methodist Church), was about five years old, and one day he had been picking cotton all day, working very hard. He looked up at me at the end of the day —and he wanted to know, do we have enough yet to pay my way to go and get the start that the church offered me? I will never forget that time, because without the offer of a scholarship I might still be working in the same cotton patch. But I want you to know, it's a long way from a community of 99 people to being your Surgeon General.

I am grateful for the support the churches in Arkansas

have given in working on health care issues. I want to single out the Reverend Bill Robinson (Little Rock) who became Chairman of our AIDS Advisory Committee when I began my work as the Health Director in Arkansas. For a long time I think Bill thought he worked for the Health Department. But because of the things he is doing, I want you to know that I changed the location of the Health Department and we are building a brand new facility, the largest one we will have in Arkansas, three blocks from his church.

I also want to mention United Methodist Bishop Richard Wilke. When we were working hard in Arkansas to get a cigarette tax passed, Bishop Wilke said, "Doctor, this is so important, and we are a part of the community, and I've got to stand up. I'll write all my churches to get behind this initiative, because it's important for the things you are trying to do."

During my tenure as a state Health Director, I remember times I was having trouble getting needed legislation passed. Once, I called the churches, and church leaders lined up around the walls, and the governor came out; and saw many of the clergy with their collars on. These church leaders had come because the legislature was holding up the Health Department budget. After the governor looked at all those ministers, and the legislators saw them all standing around the room, guess what happened? Our budget bill came quickly out of the Budget Committee.

I know that many in the religious community have been very concerned about the health issues facing our nation. We're all concerned that there are 37 million Americans who have no health insurance — people who have no place they can go for help in paying for needed treatment.

We know that in our rural communities the problem is

even greater. Many areas do not have enough doctors. We have thirty counties in Arkansas that don't even have a doctor who will deliver a baby. Most of the talk about health care reform has been primarily about how will we pay for it. But it doesn't matter how much money I have, if I don't have access to a doctor I still can't get care.

We've got to train our people how to access health care and how they ought to take care of their own health.

The churches have helped and can continue to help in many ways. For example, churches can provide transportation. We worry about how we are going to get a doctor out to serve the small rural communities; how we will assure that people get the services they require. I have told the President, "I want you to know that it's an awful lot easier to train a bus driver than it is to train a doctor." I shared this with the Secretary of Transportation, and he said, "Dr. Elders, we're going to listen to what you said." So, until we get doctors everywhere they are needed, the churches can help train bus drivers to get people to the doctors. People in our churches need to look for solutions and think together of alternative ways to address urgent needs.

I want people in the churches to know that some of the issues I've been very concerned about as Health Director in Arkansas, and will continue to be concerned about as your Surgeon General, are related to what's happening to our bright young people. I want you to know that there has been a widening of the gap between the haves and the have-nots. In 1960, one in seven children was poor. In 1990, it was one in five. For children in Arkansas (and many of the southern areas) it's one in four. If they are black or Hispanic, it's one in two. Clearly this is a major problem.

I know church people will help when they learn that we have too many children who are members of the 5-H Club. Some children are *hungry* every night, in the richest country in the world. We have 3 to 5 million children who go to bed hungry. Some children are *healthless*. Thirty-seven million Americans have no health insurance; a third of them are children. Some children are *homeless*. Out of the hundred-thousand-plus people who are homeless, a third of those are children. Some children are *hugless*— have nobody to love, nobody to care for them. If every adult would assume the responsibility for one child, we wouldn't have any children left in America who were unloved. Some children are *hopeless*. They feel there is nowhere to go, no way to get there, and that it won't make any difference what they do along the way.

I say to church leaders, we see our children out in the ocean surrounded by the sharks of drugs, alcohol, homicide, and suicide. Too often we seem willing to sit on the beach moralizing and talking about whose values are we going to teach, while our children drown.

There is a pamphlet that was put our by the department of Health in 1919 about the things we should do and how we should educate our children. In 1993 I could have it published again, and I wouldn't have had to change a word. We simply have yet to address the problems that are using up our children. I want church people to know that $66^2/_3$ percent of all of our high school seniors have tried illicit drugs. Thirty-four percent of them use drugs regularly. Fifty percent of our 12-to-17-year-olds consume more than a 6-pack of beer a week. Thirty-nine percent of our children start smoking before they leave high school. The average age of starting is 13. We know that children who smoke are 100 times more likely to use marijuana, 30 times more likely to use cocaine. And yet, when we start trying to tax the cigarette industry for what it costs — it costs us $2.17 for health care for each package of cigarettes smoked — when we start to tax it, our legislators say, "Well, Dr. Elders, we don't want to tax them out of business". Well, I want you to know, I want to tax them out of business.

I know from experience that our churches care about these issues.

We have to save the most valuable resource we'll ever have — and that's our children. We can't continue to sell them to the tobacco industry, to the liquor industry, to the gambling industry. We must save our children.

There are many statistics that sadden me. The saddest number, one that bothers me a great deal, is that only one out of five young black men will ever grown up and earn enough money to support a family. Two out of five will be lost to drugs and alcohol. One out of five will be killed by homicide. One out of five will be in prison. We have more young black men in prison than we have in college. The average cost of keeping someone in prison is $35,600 a year. We can send someone to Harvard for less than it costs to keep a person in the prison system. We've got to invest in our human capital.

Another problem that's bothering me is the marked rise in HIV, and it's rising very rapidly in our young people. One out of six of our youngsters, teenagers, will have a sexually transmitted disease every year. One out of every 250 Americans is HIV-positive. But one out of every 47 young men in high school in Washington, D.C., is HIV positive. I believe our churches can and will be places where people organize to address these needs.

Too many of our children are becoming parents before they become adults. More than a million young women —

teenagers—have children every year. Four out of ten of our young white women will become pregnant before the age of 20; 6.7 out of 10 young black women will become pregnant before they reach the age of 20; and 66 percent of them have been abused at some time in their lives. What are we going to do about it?

In Arkansas, I talked to our legislators about having rules that any young woman who became pregnant before the age of fourteen should be evaluated for possible sexual abuse. I was told, "Dr. Elders, what if she is lying?" Tell me, how can you lie when you are fourteen and pregnant? We've got to do something about it, and we know that children who have been abused are far more likely to grow up to be abusers. So we must reverse the dangerous trends that we see in our society.

We know that 80 percent of the children born to children will be poor. Only two percent will ever go to college. Only 50 percent will ever finish high school. Failure to complete high school is the most common cause of poverty in the United States. We know how to do something about this. We have the resources to do something, and yet we've not made the commitment.

People in our churches need to know that the family planning budget, of all the budgets, was less in 1992 than it was in 1982; even while we look at a marked increase in the cost of health services. So churches must begin to work with others to make a difference.

What are some of the strategies that we need to put in place to begin to bring about needed change? The first thing I feel we must do is begin to strengthen families and to strengthen family structures. To do that, we must make every child born in America a planned, wanted child.

We should have health education in our schools from

kindergarten through twelfth grade. Many people say, "Dr. Elders, let the parents do it." How can the parents do it when we didn't teach the parents? They say, "Let the church do it." You and I both know that 52 percent of the children are unchurched. They don't go to anybody's church.

My brother knows—I've always accused him, and I upset the ministers in Little Rock—I've accused them of moralizing from the pulpit and preaching to the choir. I told them they had to get out in the streets and go to work to reach the children who don't come to church on Sunday, if we're going to make a difference.

We have to begin to teach our parents how to be good parents—all of us need to be involved, and I'm included. I remember being down in the delta talking about the things we need to do, and somebody asked my son, "Kevin, what did your mother teach you?" Kevin is a wonderful son, and he didn't want to embarrass his mother before a big crowd; so he thought for a long time, but he finally said, "I don't remember my mother teaching me anything, but my daddy taught me not to get involved with anybody I didn't want to bring home." So I'm talking about you and me when I say that we've just not taught our parents how to deal with these issues. We have to begin to teach our young males responsibility. We've allowed them to walk around and donate sperm and feel that was equivalent to being a father. We have to teach them how to be responsible.

We have to offer all of our young people hope of going to college, so they will be good students and good citizens. All children should be provided an opportunity to go to college whether or not their parents can afford it. It is far cheaper to pay for college than it is to pay for prison.

I have said many times that we should make sure that

all Americans have universal access to health care. Every person accused of a crime has a constitutional right to be represented by a lawyer; why don't we feel that people who are sick have a right to have a doctor? We have to focus on prevention. We must be allowed to intervene to educate and help people, and we must feel that we can get away with intervening. We have acted in our society as if everything were disposable, even our children. But we have to prevent many of the problems that we see, and we must teach our people how to be responsible for their own health care if we are ever going to make a significant difference.

Certainly our churches want to be effective in building a hope-filled future for our children. To do so, we must alleviate the causes of poverty which breed suffering and hopelessness.

Think about the word *alleviate* with me. For each of the letters, I have chosen special words so we won't forget what we must do.

For the first letter *a* in **alleviate**, we have to be *aware* of the problems that are affecting our communities. If we aren't aware of something, we can't do anything about it. We must open up our eyes and our ears, and begin to look, to listen, and to use all our senses to increase our awareness. But I don't want you to stop there. Just being aware is not enough. We have to become advocates for the solutions to these problems. The we have to develop action plans that fit our own communities if we are going to make a difference.

For the first *l* in **alleviate**, I chose the word **leadership**. We must step out and be willing to lead. Too many of us go out and find which way the wind is blowing and jump out in front. We have to be the headlights; we have been the taillights too long. Our churches already have credibility; they have both human resources and building resources. Now we should reach out and get everybody involved.

For the next *l*, I like the word *linkages*. Churches have lots of linkages, through your community, linkages with the places people work, linkages with other organizations, linkages that connect people all over this country. We can change what needs to be changed if we choose to do so. We can make sure we have a health care system in America, and we don't have to accept it when people say, "We don't have the money." Think about what we already spend. We spend 33 million dollars an hour on national defense. We spend 23 million dollars an hour to service the national debt. We spend 8 million dollars an hour bailing out the failed savings and loan institutions, but we spend only 2.3 million dollars on health care and our children. So it is quite simply a matter of how we choose to spend our money.

Next is *e*, for *educate*. He have to *educate*. We have to educate ourselves. We have to educate our policy makers. We have to educate our parishioners. We have to educate our community about the problems we must face. We have to educate those who teach in our schools. As you know, I have been a strong proponent of comprehensive school-based health services. Twenty percent of our population is in school every day. Many say, "Oh, but Dr. Elders, we can't have those school-based clinics because they might end up doing an abortion." Well, there has never been a woman who needed an abortion who was not already pregnant. In my work I have been about preventing pregnancies; I have never been about abortion. We should stop worrying about the abortion issue, and worry more about preventing pregnancies.

For the *v*, church members and clergy must provide the *voice* and the *vision* for the poor and the powerless. If our churches won't do it, who will?

I stands for invest. We must invest in the most valuable resource we have—our people. If we don't invest in our people, we are destined to be burdened with a large salvage operation.

The second *a* is for *alliances*. We have to form alliances with everybody. Let's form alliances with other churches; with organizations we haven't spoken to before. Together we can do what we need to do to make a difference.

To borrow one of my brother's lines; in order to get it done we have to be committed. We have to make the commitment if we want to get the job done of building a hope-filled future. What are the tools of commitment? There are three Ts: We have to give our *time*, we have to give of our *talents*, and yes, we have to give of our *treasures*.

For the last *e* in *alleviate* I have chosen the word *empower*. We have to empower the church to become a hospital for sinners, rather than a haven for the saved. We have to begin to do these things so that we can make a difference. We can't keep putting on a bandage when we need major surgery. If we are going to reform our health care system, we have to do more than offer rhetoric.

I know that the leaders and members of our churches have been working hard. As your Surgeon General, I want you to know that I don't mind being the lighting rod, but I have to know—and I do know—that people in churches across America will be the thunder I hear, cheering me on.

I want to share with you a saying of Bishop Kenneth Hicks, former United Methodist Bishop for the Arkansas

70

Area. He said, "When you are dancing with the bear, you can't get tired and sit down; you wait until the bear gets tired, and then you sit down." We need to work side by side to bring together a lot of new partners who will cut in and make sure that we can keep that bear busy!

What is the Role of Our Churches?

How can we answer the call of the Spirit to alleviate human suffering in these challenging times?

- We have to admit that we can't do it alone.
- We have to get everyone involved. The churches, the schools, our businesses—we all must become involved if we are going to make a difference we can see. Many of us have been so busy attending to maintenance tasks that we have forgotten our mission. Our mission is to make sure that all of our people reach their full potential. I know that we in America's churches are willing to do what our communities need done.
- We must remind ourselves that we are doers, so we have to get about the business of getting to work and achieving results.

I hope you will remind me, as I will remind you, "When you are dancing with the bear, you can't get tired and sit down; you wait until the bear gets tired, and then you sit down."

NINE

The Religious And Moral Value-Orientation Of Dr. Elders

"Where there is no vision the people perish ..." Proverbs 29:18, King James Version.

As her brother and pastor, I have shared many conversations with Dr. Elders about the church's role as moral agent for the Lord. Dr. Elders believes that today's church must renew its understanding of its prophetic call if it is going to address the social, political and economic challenges of our changing society.

The church, she says, "needs to be in position to understand and interpret to persons of society who are experiencing social, political and economic turmoil." Of course, I believe the prophetic call to which Dr. Elders made reference is religious rather than social, political or economic. But the more she has shared with me, the more I am moved to try to visualize her point.

Dr. Elders believes a pastor cannot act as a moral agent if he or she is too far outside the household of faith, and there deeply into the problems of the world. If found in this situation, "then he or she has lost connection with the unique environment of the church and cannot be effective," she says. It is this connection which enables the pastor to interface with the community as moral agent and gap filler. One cannot fulfill the call to ministry as moral agent and teacher unless one is standing in the gap; one cannot fulfill moral responsibility scripturally by being so far into the church camp that he or she can only see the problems of society from a distance," she said. I asked if she was also saying that to stand in the gap as moral agent, the pastor must experience an encounter with a suffering God. For it is only in conversion and commitment to follow a suffering God that the pastor can understand the plight of those wounded by transgressions of a sinful people. She complimented me on my "ministerial insight .."

Thus, the pastor must interface with church and society if he or she is to fulfill the role of moral agent. Many times, this role is uncomfortable but is the only position to which a pastor is called.

Dr. Elders believes that the church, as we know it, has either lost or never had the vision which allows both a multi-cultural and pluralistic society. The church, as we know it, is divided along racial, gender, class and economic lines and cannot fulfill the divine mission entrusted to it, that of saving and winning the world for Christ. God cannot be divided into a liberal or conservative deity. John 4:24, King James Version, tells us that, "God is a spirit and they that worship him must worship in spirit and truth."

The profound problem of a racially divided pluralistic society is to cultivate respect for the viability and integrity of every group's experience. To interpret pluralistic circumstances with a religious tradition influenced by only one part of the plurality often leaves no ability to see the vision of a multi-cultural and pluralistic society.

In our society, what we think is often determined by where it is that we do our thinking. Perhaps that is why Dr. Elders spent thirty years in hospitals as a doctor and teacher without speaking out on many of the social ills and wrongs of our society. Her critics may ask, "If you are so concerned about the children, why didn't you speak out earlier? Why did you not say something over the past thirty years?" Her answer is complex and yet, very simple. "What we think is determined almost one hundred per cent by where it is we do our thinking."

For example, we know that we have been asking the wrong questions about domestic violence for years. We know the real question involves helping women leave abusive situations. A disturbing fact which impedes our motivation to resolve the problem of domestic violence is that so often the abuser is a well respected member of society. Therefore, we go on asking ourselves why abused women don't just leave.

Dr. Elders did what most doctors do. I believe doctors spend ninety percent of their time thinking about treatment and only ten percent of their time thinking about prevention. I think there is now some degree of change in this behavior. After becoming Director of The Arkansas Department of Health, it did not take Dr. Elders long to see that it is incumbent upon all of us to change our attitude toward public health and to think more about prevention.

Dr. Elders said, "The health of our nation is inextricably entwined with the health of our citizens. To meet the multifaceted challenges of the twenty-first century, we must visualize, conceptualize and actualize a plan for a healthy America." All in all, Dr. Elders seems to feel that the church needs a "reality slap" if we are to move its leadership toward consideration of the past when making plans for the future.

Figuratively speaking, we are all provided two maps we

can follow in life. One map is drawn based on the way things really are — reality. Generally, we just accept the points of this map as being accurate — the way things are. On the other hand, the second map is drawn based on the way we believe things ought to be — values. For the most part, our attitudes and behaviors are shaped by the values map. Many of us assume that the way we perceive things is the right way. We also know that we should not assume.

Many major inventions or scientific breakthroughs came with a break from tradition. Dr. Elders believes that today's problems of drug abuse, violence and teen pregnancy we face cannot be resolved with traditional thinking. Instead, she believes we must get out of the box, reassess our thinking and change when necessary. This does not mean that she advocates anti-religious, immoral, unethical or illegal solutions. She wishes we could understand that her philosophies are a means to expand our thinking and actions beyond the point where these problems grow to the crisis stage.

We Must Visualize

We must visualize a health care program that will produce a healthy America. If we can't visualize such a program, then how can we design it? Dr. Elders, in her crusade for an improved quality of life for all Americans, calls for major surgery on our attitude toward public health. To say it another way, she thinks that as a nation we must visualize the individual and family benefits of teaching comprehensive health education in our schools from grades K to 12.

The objective of this visualization is to see how to meet a

need God tells us must be met. Dr. Elders explains that we must learn the difference between a vision and a dream. To her, a vision is always clear; if not, the call is not heard. This point is made clear in the Bible in what is often referred to as the "Macedonian call," which leads one to believe that a vision is rooted in faith. Before the Lord can turn us, He first has to stop us. The Bible tells us that Paul was stopped on his journey to Asia by the Holy Ghost so God could use him in some other place.

In the Book of Acts, Chapter 16, Verses 9, 10, (King James Version), we are told of Paul's Macedonian Vision: "And avision appeared to Paul in the night; There stood a man of Macedonia, and prayed him, saying, Come over into Macedonia, and help us. And after he had seen the vision, immediately we endeavored to go into Macedonia, assuredly gathering that the Lord had called us to preach the gospel unto them ... "

At times, I feel that going to the Arkansas Department of Health was Dr. Elder's "Macedonian call," because her vision now seems clear. If the vision is clear, the call to serve for justice, love and mercy truly was heard by the recipients. However, trouble may follow for the hearer; this can be especially true when the hearer meets with the sleepers and dreamers of society. Due to the nature of each, there is likely to be some degree of conflict between the visionaries and the dreamers; between the prophets and the evangelists, between the liberals and conservatives; and yes, between Elders and some religious politicians.

The problem with the dreamers of society is that they never seem to wake up! Real vision calls for seeing and believing. Dreams are more passive, visions more active. While her initial focus was teaching medical students, Dr.

Elders entered a new realm of seeing and believing when she began helping Arkansans find solutions to public health problems. Frequently, Dr. Elders has said, "Most of us were taught as young children that an ounce of prevention is worth a pound of cure." In addition, she has stated that, "In America, we spend almost thirteen percent of the gross national product on medical costs, but less than three percent of that amount goes for prevention initiatives and programs." One study shows that more than one third of the American population is without any health insurance.

Dr. Elders interprets her "Macedonian call" as a mandate to work toward health care protection for every American. Her vision for a healthy America involves preventing chronic and infectious diseases such as AIDS, tuberculosis, cancer, hypertension, heart disease; reducing infant morbidity and mortality; eliminating the disparity in health problems and care between minorities and non-minorities; improving health care for all women; providing better health for the elderly; reducing, if not eradicating, drug abuse and violence, and reducing the incidence of teenage pregnancy.

We Must Conceptualize

Americans are called to conceptualize a new health care plan, to map out a plan that addresses the health care needs of all Americans. We must come together and map out the who, what, how, when, and where of a comprehensive plan. We must decide where we are going with health care reform, and estimate the costs in realistic terms. The process of this conceptualization must be rooted in faith, and the faith must be rooted in prayer and reality. In estimating the cost, we must remember the biblical advice,

"For which of you, intending to build a tower, sitteth not down first, and counteth the cost, whether he have sufficient to finish it?" (Luke 14:28, King James Version)

We all know that nothing is more frustrating than starting a project and lacking sufficient resources and skills to complete it. We witness such frustration in the effort of the Clinton administration to draw up an acceptable health care plan, which is still on the drawing board nearly four years later.

Health care for every American is not beyond the resources, skills and capacities of our country as some people would have us believe. The first obstacle we must overcome is the lack of vision. We must visualize a plan before we can conceptualize the blueprint and strategies needed to implement the vision. Next, we must have the will and resolve to make it happen.

Dr. Elders has said many times, "If we want to help our nation remain strong and continue to produce leaders of the world, we had better conceptualize a plan to save our future — the children." She believes our future depends on the health and education of our children. I have heard her say many times, "Too many children in one of the richest countries in the world are hungry, homeless, helpless, hugless and hopeless." She laments, "Thus, the children, who are our only hope for the future, are hanging by a very thin thread as far as hope for a healthy future."

"Therefore," she says, "until we address the problems in our society which have resulted in children being poorly housed or homeless, poorly fed, educated and lacking adequate health care, we will continue to hand out band aids when what the patients need is major surgery." The major surgery to which she refers has to do with the way we deal with health care in America. Her message is that with the present strategies for public health, "We aren't paying for health care, we are paying for dying care!" She believes we must become more conscious of health care prevention if we hope to heal our health care ills.

To accomplish what Dr. Elders advocates means we must change our attitude and behavior concerning dying care and start thinking about prevention based on health care support. We must change our conceptualization of what health care means. Health care was never meant to be abused and misused, and many times, abuse of insurance is driving companies out of business. There has to be a cap on the services which any of us can expect to receive. Of course, we understand that there are no unlimited supplies. This is true of the air we breathe. If we pollute the air, somewhere down the line we suffer the consequences.

The bottom line is we must change our attitude and behavior to implement more health care prevention programs. The choice to prolong life at any cost has been perpetuated by the notion that we can have anything we can afford. The notion that doctors can cure us of anything is a dream that has turned into a nightmare for thousands of patients. We are told that too much tobacco, alcohol, food, lack of exercise and sleep are bad for our health. Yet, millions of us see these warnings as applicable to other people and not intended for us. Unfortunately, the day of judgment comes when we find that our doctor cannot provide a cure. Then, we ask ourselves why we did not heed the warning. This is why, on that so-called "day of judgment," many of us will spend most of our time looking back instead of looking forward to a new life.

We Must Actualize

As Americans, we are called to actualize a new health care plan that provides for all: a vehicle that every American can utilize to access health care services. Actualization can be likened to building a bridge that will bridge the present gaps in our health care system. The bridge (new health care plan) must be strong enough to support both those who contribute their share and even those unable to contribute.

I think that to develop our new health care bridge, it would be wise to consider the advice of an engineer. An engineer who builds bridges once said, "Before I start to build a bridge, I have to consider three loads the bridge must bear. The first is the dead load, the weight of the bridge itself. The second is the live load, the weight of all the traffic the bridge must bear. The third is the wind load, the elements of nature and all the circumstances beyond our control."

When we look at all the different needs of our citizenry, we should heed the advice of the bridge engineer. Why? Because when we consider building our comprehensive health care bridge, we must take into consideration that forty-three million Americans either don't have, or can't afford, health insurance. This is a growing situation that must be considered when we actualize a new health care plan.

As I ponder the health care situation, I am reminded of a little rhyme that I remember from my childhood that goes like this:

A bridge engineer, Mr. Trumpet,
Built a bridge for the good River Bumppet,
A mistake in the plan left a gap in the span,
But he said, "They'll just have to jump it!"

It would seem that our lawmakers are saying to us that we'll just have to jump it! But how can we keep jumping over the fact that one million American families seek health care every year and are turned away for the lack of ability to pay? How do we continue to jump over the fact that another 14 or 15 million do not look for health care because they know they can't afford it? How can we continue to ignore the fact that infant mortality in the United States is higher than in sixteen other industrialized countries? In addition, perhaps we need to declare a state of emergency just to address the basic health care needs of children. American children are now less healthy, less educated and less motivated than children in many other industrialized countries.

Dr. Elders has stated that if we expect to develop strong, educated and motivated leadership for our future, we had better actualize a comprehensive, prevention based health care plan. After all, she says, "Until we address the problems in society which have resulted in children being poorly fed, educated, motivated and without adequate prenatal and neonatal care, we lack the vision to conceptualize, actualize and build the vehicle by which we can deliver our children a safe and healthy future."

TEN

On Practicing What We Preach
How Can the Christian Church Make a Difference?

We all know that the basic role of the Christian Church is to carry out "the great commission," to go into all the world and win souls for Jesus Christ, to make a caring and safe environment-consistent with the principle of love. But how do we make this theological concept real? How do we put hands and feet on the gospel in order to make a tangible difference in the world. How can the Church, in all its roles, play a part in encouraging our government, indeed, our entire nation, to visualize, conceptualize and actualize a health care plan by which we can all benefit?

If our nation is to turn the tide of rising poverty, crime, disease and death, it will take all of us working together. One of the best vehicles for making a positive social change is the one institution that has the potential to reach millions and that has as its primary mission to love all and serve the world. The Christian community lives by the values of faith, hope and love as demonstrated by Jesus Christ. Based on these values, the Church is well positioned to serve as a conduit for networking among the government, school systems, businesses and communities. The Church is particularly well suited to empower individuals as agents of change in various communities.

There are those who feel the Church's role now, and in the new century, is to give support to people in the midst of swift and major transition, even as they view the church as suffering from "spiritual asphyxiation." I disagree. Surely the Church can do more to lend support to the needy from all levels of society. Surely the Church can do something to direct the course of the transition our society is experiencing. Surely the Church is about helping to promote health and insuring the welfare of all people, regardless of race, creed or economic position. Our task is to engage in a serious dialogue between the Church and the needs and concerns of our nation in order to develop a plan to make our country stronger and healthier. Dr. Elders and I have discussed, at length, what may be the role of the Church in the development of a viable health care plan. Dr. Elders believes that the Church should become more involved in ministries which help to restore basic family values of faith, hope, love, self-respect, self-esteem, self-confidence, honesty, trust and healthy minds, souls and bodies. I have attempted to recapture some of the discussions we have had in the pages that follow.

Reverend Jones:

> Joycelyn, you are always saying the church should be doing more in helping to devise a viable, universal public health care plan. You have said many times that in our country, while every citizen has a right to an attorney, every citizen should have a right to a doctor. So what would you have the churches do?

Dr. Elders:

> The first question the Church must ask is: "Does everyone have a right to health care?" If not, why not. If so, how much health care? After this discussion, the churches

could work through their members and community organizations and, perhaps, in some cases, partnerships to establish the following kinds of programs to promote healthy lifestyles:

1. Begin church sponsored older adult care programs to offer families a respite from their care-giving duties — such programs might also afford the elderly opportunities to socialize with others through games, crafts, music, exercises and other activities

2. Initiate church sponsored Men Against Destruction/Defending Against Drugs and Social Disorder (Mad Dad) chapters, with emphasis on counseling troubled youngsters, removing graffiti from neighborhoods and establishing neighborhood patrols

3. Sponsor dialogues where the Clergy could speak about health issues and support school health education.

4. Work to dispel the attitude of some Christians who believe they are the only custodians and interpreters of God's law and will not support comprehensive health education in public schools. We must all work together for health is not an isolated issue. A sick person affects the health of all of us.

5. Institute viable programs for teaching and assisting young mothers in caring for infants and children.

6. Establish ways to work through members and community organizations to recapture our communities from drugs dealers and criminals by supporting Church based recovery programs and counseling in more churches.

7. Declare the churches safe sanctuaries for teen mothers who live in dangerous neighborhoods besieged by gangs, drugs and violence by providing supportive services and counseling.

8. Start community development centers where teen parents can receive information about parenting skills, sex education, drug abuse and social ills, plus get immunizaation shots for their children.

9. Help sponsor more alternative schools for troubled youths.

10. Compile role model resource banks to help motivate troubled youths as they make a commitment to change - each local church could adopt an issue, develop expertise in the field, and could be called upon to serve a wide geographic area.

11. Host support groups/victim assistance programs for victims of violence

12. Establish youth revival of hope centers to comprehensively address the many

health care concerns for a geographic area.

13. Support church/community foster care, as well as group homes for those youths who cannot be placed because of disabilities and other circumstances.

14. Start crime prevention centers to facilitate values and attitudes which seem to have made violence so common in our society

15. Host forums where community members can discuss the challenges of living and coping in the new century, learn the biblical ethic, "love thy neighbor as thyself," and determine how to obtain peace through moral strength

Dr. Elders:

From your perspective as a minister, what are some of the major challenges the church must deal with to prepare communities to build a public health plan?

Reverend Jones:

Our challenges include efforts to help people understand the following list of topics:

1. The theological implications of drugs, alcohol, violence, sex, teen pregnancies and 12-step programs such as AA/NA.

2. The moral, economic and spiritual needs

of families

3. The theological, moral, social and economic costs of racism

4. The needs of those suffering from loneliness caused by death, divorce, single life, etc.

5. The plight of women in our society

6. The meaning of a Christ-centered life - The church's moral standards must be above those of the secular world

7. The ways to make the church a place of healing, where people can share their pain and suffering and receive comfort and assurance

8. The need to establish church reading/study centers, where people can read, study and discuss the Bible

9. The role of ecumenical prison ministries which assist inmates released from prison

10. The crisis of teen suicide and homicide, and the American problems of guns and violence

11. The need to instill prevention as part of our culture and way of thinking-we need to be active, rather than reactive

12. The vision and power that God has given the church, His "light of the world and salt of the earth" - The church should be a catalyst, establishing communities of Shalom through the world

13. Conflict resolution techniques

14. The potential inherent in evils, principalities and powers

15. The special needs of the culturally disenfranchised - those who have been forced to give up their own cultures and adapt cultures foreign to them

Dr. Elders:

So, you do agree the church has broad roles to play in developing a viable public health care plan?

Reverend Jones:

Precisely, the church has a major role to play, that of educating Americans to apply God's word when distributing resources, care and services. I think this is what has been missing in the design of our programs: the demonstration of real love for one another and for God. I think the church must see to it that what we preach becomes what we practice, that we "walk the walk" as well as of "talk the talk."

How Can the Christian Church Make a Difference?

The question for the Church, it seems to me, is how we keep the commandment -- given over and over again in the scriptures, "love your neighbor as yourself?" This is the key for the church, if we are to make any real difference in the needs of our world, where the health and welfare of our country is concerned

Christianity must become a kind of lifestyle that is truly Christlike, when we live as Jesus lived. If we examine Jesus' life, and take it as the archetype for Christian life, we clearly see that we must be constantly about reaching out and touching people where their needs are.

Jesus was always reaching out to those around him in need: sinners, tax collectors, women, children, the sick, the disenfranchised. What he did was not always popular with the institutional religion of the day. He didn't fit into any of the stereotypical roles of religious teacher. Likewise the church must be bold today. We must move beyond the strictures of "the way we've always done it" in the institutional church and take chances with new ways of reaching out to the "sinners, tax collectors, women children, sick and disenfranchised" of our day. We must move beyond the view of the church as a "sacred society" with a mission only to protect our way of life. We must get beyond the stance that "others are not deserving" of what the church has to offer. We must spend less time worrying about which groups' lifestyles we disapprove of and more time worrying about how the gospel can be made real in everyone's life.

If the institutional church spent more time living as Jesus did, reaching out to people in need, touching people where they hurt, providing tangible relief for their pain, and less time organizing Mickey Mouse boycotts, our world would be a better place.

The story in Mark chapter 2 (2:1-5; 11-12) tells about some people who were so insistent upon getting their sick friend into a crowded house where Jesus was ministering that they climbed up, pulled back part of the roof and lowered him into the room at Jesus' feet. This is the kind of effort we need to be expending for our world today. It is time for us to take the roof off the institutional church as we know it, shake things up a bit and bring the wounded, weary world into the healing power of the church.

It is time for the church to stop "being" Christian and start "doing" Christianity, become "doers of the word, not hearers only (James 1:22). There are a multitude of ways we can begin to make a difference for the health and welfare of our country. Some churches may already be doing many of these things. If so, then those churches may need to find other ways to reach out. Many churches are doing none of these things. If that is the case, they need to be prodded into service of the gospel they profess to proclaim.

This list is by no means exhaustive, merely some ideas for ways the church can start to do more about "loving our neighbors."

1. Programs to reach the homeless
2. Big Brothers/Big Sisters programs
3. Seminars in celebrating diversity, becoming as comfortable with others as we are with ourselves, moving beyond stereotypes, raising the level of what we will tolerate from others
4. Program initiatives, training and exploring race relations, which are the root problems of power,

powerlessness and fear
5. Volunteers In Mission projects
6. Food pantries
7. Prayer vigils to reach out with compassion to persons in need
8. Groups to call on the sick and homebound
9. Counseling services-physical, emotional care and support
10. Treatment programs, support groups for addictions
11. Scholarship assistance for college students
12. A response team to local disasters-emergency housing, financial aid, utilities, medicine, clothing and shelter
13. Child care scholarships for young mothers
14. Tutoring services for school children
15. Volunteers to deliver Meals on Wheels
16. Teams to provide transportation to doctor appointments for older persons or those without any other form of transportation
17. HOSPICE volunteers
18. RAIN (AIDS ministry) volunteers
19. Clothing thrift shops
20. Recycling programs
21. Groups to "glean" fields of fruits and vegetables for low-income families
22. Walk-a-thons, or other fund-raisers for mission and outreach
23. Sponsor health fairs, mission fairs, education fairs, etc.
24. Donate canning equipment to low-income families
25. Support Heifer Project International, UMCOR initiatives and other designated programs which provide assistance to needy families
26. Work teams to improve low-income housing
27. Support groups like Habitat for Humanity
28. Organize voter registration drives

29. Workshops on AIDS, Youth Crime, Addiction, Education, Economic Empowerment, Death/Dying, Multicultural Social Change
30. Support programs dedicated to the prevention of alcohol, tobacco and other drugs
31. Host Alcoholics Anonymous, AlAnon, CODA and other twelve step recovery groups
32. Workshops for youth on how to handle peer pressure
33. Mentoring programs targeting junior high students
34. Workshops on alternatives to violence and gangs
35. After-school programs for children and youth
36. Evening and late night programs to keep kids off the streets
37. Prison ministry

The bottom line for the church today is that we must be about proclaiming with our lips and our lives a message of love. The crime, violence, addiction and other social horrors today are symptoms of a society that is crying out for love, acceptance and discipline. Like the small child who "acts out" to gain attention, there are millions crying out in negative ways today. The church has the answer to this core problem - "God so loved the world" (John 3:16). Our children, youth, young adults are crying out for someone to give them the attention and love that everyone deserves, to give them the order and discipline that everyone needs. It is apparent when I look at what is happening in our prisons today, there are hordes of people crying out for order and discipline. When I see the way young black men in our prisons are turning to the Islamic faith, I realize that what they need is order, discipline and structure in their lives. This is what they are finding in Islam. Then I must ask myself, why can't the Christian faith offer the same sort of order and discipline and structure?

The key, I believe, is for us to put all our energy into making the church an active institution, not a reactive one, to making the message of the gospel real in people's lives, teaching them to actively live Christlike lives. It is an old cliche, "to practice what you preach," but it is precisely what our world needs. The health and welfare of our country depends on it. This has been Dr. Elder's message and it is my message. It must become the message of the church, the action of the church, the everyday way of life for the church. We must remember the eleventh commandment, the one I learned from the people I grew up around, "thou shalt not quit." I learned this from people who made a way out of no way, people who believed that with God all things are possible. God can enable us to do far more than we can ever imagine. The key is that we must be willing to do. If the church is to make a difference, we must get to work living out the message of love that is uniquely ours.

ELEVEN
Concluding Reflections
Who Needs Family Values

Chester R. Jones

Dr. Elders has said many times that "we see our children out in the ocean surrounded by the sharks of drugs, alcohol, teenage pregnancy, homicide, and suicide, and we are sitting on the beach moralizing and talking about whose values are going to be taught, while our children drown." I had heard my sister make this statement many times   before I got up enough nerve to ask her what she meant by it. I somehow had a sneaky feeling that after coming to hear her younger brother preach for fifty-two straight weeks, she could be talking about me. I did not want to believe it.

After I first moved back to Arkansas to pastor a church, my wife, Valarie, and I ate dinner with my sister and brother-in-law, Coach Elders, every Sunday. One Sunday I asked her, "Joycelyn, who are these people on the beach moralizing and talking about whose values they are going to teach, while our children drown?" She said to me, "You, and many other ministers I know who just stand in the pulpit and moralize about what people should not do!" Then she said something that hurt me at the time but that I later understood: "You should be out in the street working and ministering where the people with real needs are. The church," she said, "needs to move from the amen corner to the street corner, where the people I am talking about are."

Who needs family values? Dr. Elders feels that the church should be more involved in ministries to help restore basic family values of self-confidence, self-respect, self-esteem, honesty, trust, faith, hope, and love.

Some people have criticized my sister because they feel that school-based clinics will turn into condom clinics and not teach young people to say *no*. However, on the other hand, some feel that clinics can make parents and teachers more aware of the need to teach abstinence as the real value that everyone should follow before marriage.

I am a United Methodist district superintendent. I know that every pastor in my district teaches and preaches that God's design for sex is only within marriage. We preach that God created sex to confirm a lifelong union between two married people. To preach any other gospel would lead to a state of progressive moral decay in our Christian, biblically based value system. I tell my sister that the parents, the church, and the school—the early care-givers to most children I come in contact with—must play major roles in passing on our values to children.

But my sister challenges me: "What about the 52 percent of the people in this country who are unchurched and may not be a part of a value system that holds to a biblically based marriage? What about children who are born to teenagers outside the marriage bond?"

What about the young mother or child who has been abused, physically or sexually? What about the young child that is born HIV+? What about the young teenager who commits suicide? What about an inter-racial marriage? What about the teenager who is sexually active? What about divorced parents? What about the person who faces a terminal illness?

She raises difficult questions with me, as her longtime pastor, and with the church: "Is there no gospel in the church for unwed teenagers and women who get pregnant and choose to have an abortion? Will the church not be a father to the child out of wedlock? Will the church not be a friend to the teenager who chooses to have an abortion?" After all, we preach that Jesus is a friend to sinners and a father to the fatherless. Did Jesus come to save the whole world, or just the church-approved membership list? Did not the Master say, "Whosoever will" may come, not whosover is approved?

It has not been easy to be Dr. Elder's pastor and brother. I feel that sometimes she must stay awake all night to come up with these questions. However, I must admit, that as a pastor, I splend a great deal of my time answering questions that no one is asking. Finally, I am grateful that there is only one Joycelyn Elders in our family. I will venture to say, God blessed America by having only one like her in the country.

TO BE PUBLISHED

The following is taken from my book on Religious Humor From the Black Tradition, which will be published in November of 1998.

The story is told of two brothers from the state of Arkansas, Zeke and Zed, who were cotton farmers. After a couple of bad crop years their farm went into foreclosure and was auctioned. They only had one old mule left after the farm was sold. They were both sad and asked the auctioneer if he knew where they may find some work. He said, "I am not sure, but I heard Southwest Airlines had an office in Little Rock, and was hiring."

So, Zeke and Zed got on their old mule and rode up the highway from down in the Delta to the employment office of Southwest Airlines. They arrived early on a Monday morning. When the employment office opened, Zeke and Zed were the first in line. They had to decide which one would go in first. Zed told Zeke since he was the oldest brother, he should go first.

So Zeke went and knocked on the door and the personnel director said, "Come in and have a seat." After the preliminary questions he asked Zeke, "What are your skills?" Zeke said, "I am a pilot." The personnel director said, "Wonderful,- we can use some good pilots at this airlines, and we will pay you $80,000 a year. Now just sign this contract and come back in a week and take our refresher training for all new pilots."

Zeke left the office and went out and told his brother, "Zed, I did not know it would be that easy. I just got a job making $80,000 a year as a pilot."

His younger brother Zed let out a shout, "Woo-pe, let me go in and see what I can do." Zed knocked on the door and the personnel director said, "Come in and have a seat." After the preliminaries, the personnel director said to Zed, "What are your skills?" He said, "I am a woodcutter." The personnel director said, "A woodcutter! What makes you think you can get a job at this great up and coming airline as a woodcutter?"

He said, "Well, you just gave my brother a job."

He said, "Yes, but your brother is a pilot."

Zed said, "But he can't pile-it until I cut it!"

Reverend Jones is the author of two other books, *"Dancing with the Bear"* and *"Dancing with Little Teddy."* Request books from #1 Longmeadow, Pine Bluff, AR 71603. Also, copies of *"From Sharecropper's Daughter to Surgeon General of the United States of America,"* by Dr. Joycelyn Elders and David Chanoff can be ordered from the same address.

870-534-1738